# Better Physician Writing and Speaking Skills

Improving Communication, Grant Writing
and Chances for Publication

# Better Physician Writing and Speaking Skills

## Improving Communication, Grant Writing and Chances for Publication

**John Gartland, MD**
*James Edwards Professor, Emeritus, Orthopaedic Surgery*
*University Medical Editor*
*Jefferson Medical College of Thomas Jefferson University*
*Philadelphia, PA*

Radcliffe Publishing
Oxford • Seattle

MT

**Radcliffe Publishing Ltd**
18 Marcham Road
Abingdon
Oxon OX14 1AA
United Kingdom

**www.radcliffe-oxford.com**
Electronic catalogue and worldwide online ordering facility.

---

British Library Cataloguing in Publication Data

A catalogue record for this book is available from the British Library.

ISBN-10: 1 84619 174 2
ISBN-13: 978 1 84619 174 9

Typeset by Anne Joshua & Associates, Oxford, UK
Printed and bound by Biddles Ltd, King's Lynn, Norfolk, UK

2|1|08

Dedicated to the memory of
William Russell MacAusland Jr, MD,
superb physician and friend

# Contents

# Preface

The medical profession regards good interpersonal skills, good communication skills and good writing skills as necessary and desirable attributes for all physicians to possess. The ability to interact in a positive manner with all patients is also a long-established goal of effective medical practice and medical education. Despite its acknowledged professional importance, helping medical students to attain proficiency in these medical skills appears to be given little prominence in the traditional period of medical education when contrasted with the emphasis placed on teaching new medical treatment developments. As a consequence, medical schools now tend to produce some medical graduates who are inclined to display a disproportionate lack of balance between caring and curing. Admittedly, medical knowledge and clinical skills are the cornerstones of good patient care, but what needs to be emphasized to all physicians is that the catalysts for transforming good patient care into good and effective patient care are the communication and interpersonal skills of the treating physician.

The ability to write and speak clearly and logically about medical matters is an important and desirable skill for all physicians to work hard to master. A vital element of effective medical communication, be it written or spoken, is clarity in the presented message, so that there is no possibility that either the reader or the listener will misinterpret or misunderstand the presented message. However, regularly mentioned criticisms of physicians' written and spoken messages point to a distinct lack of clarity in those messages. Developing acceptable writing and speaking skills, then, should be major goals for all physicians to attempt to attain, because the very nature of the medical profession is such that few physicians can escape the need to speak and write in their professional careers. I share with you in this book concepts and strategies relating to medical writing, medical speaking and patient communication skills that have worked well for me over a long academic medical career. My hope is that these suggested communication and writing strategies will work as well for you as they have for me over many years.

John J Gartland, MD
*November 2006*

# About the Author

John J Gartland, **AB, MD** is Board certified in orthopaedic surgery, and served as the James Edwards Professor of Orthopaedic Surgery and the Department Chairman, Jefferson Medical College of Thomas Jefferson University, Philadelphia, PA, from 1970 to 1985. He is the author of 135 published medical articles and four orthopaedic text-books. He is now Medical Editor at Thomas Jefferson University, Philadelphia, PA.

Chapter 1

# Physician Writing and Speaking Skills

Today, perhaps more than ever before, physicians need to improve their image in the eyes of the public. Some professional observers of the present medical care scene believe that today's physicians seem more interested in the number of patients they can shuttle through their offices than they are in the number of patient cures they can provide. Today's physicians are not regarded as good communicators by most patients. But it was not always that way.

During the nineteenth century the writer, Robert Louis Stevenson, described physicians as the flower of civilization, and it is instructive to speculate why physicians of that century may have deserved such an accolade. During Stevenson's time medical science was minimal, medical technology was primitive, and diseases were rampant and frequently fatal. Yet, despite these almost overwhelming obstacles, physicians cared for patients with the limited resources available to them at the time. Their most potent weapon proved to be their ability to inspire their patients' trust and confidence. This element of charismatic authority, which was wielded in a positive manner by physicians of those days, encouraged patients to help and heal themselves. For this, more than for their rather primitive medical skills, these physicians were regarded as humanitarians and, as such, were accorded Stevenson's floral tribute. However, from the time when Stevenson bestowed this praise on physicians to the present time, his floral tribute seems to have wilted.

Society now tends to believe that today's medical practitioners have, to a varying degree, lost sight of this idealism and professionalism, and have become to some extent a profession whose primary goal seems to be professional self-interest and financial return rather than the welfare of their patients. A lack of a warm, caring attitude of physicians toward their patients, coupled with their perceived overemphasis on the technological aspects of medical care, are the reasons most frequently given by society to justify their present assessment of physicians in general. Society now believes that physicians are well enough educated to address the health problems of patients and the treatment of specific disease states, but it also suspects that many present-day physicians are unable to deal with the patient as a person. Present-day society tends to believe that today's physicians are poorly educated for providing the kind of emotional support that a patient often desperately needs when faced with a poor medical outcome.

In defense of physicians, however, it must be admitted that the current environment of medical practice in this country is unsettled because of interactions between the different objectives being pursued by the federal government in order to contain medical costs. Despite having the highest per capita expenditure in the world for health and medical care, the United States has neither the equity in access to health services nor the highest level of health compared with other developed countries. This has led to frequent disagreements between the medical profession, society and the government about how to contain the rising costs of providing health care in this country.[1] Attempting to gain control over the continuing escalation of health care costs has become a major focus of this country's national health policy, as the available financial resources do have finite limits. These limits relate to the large federal deficit that is currently causing concern among the citizens of this country, which to a certain extent limits the amount of money available for improving the country's present health care system.

Society has become increasingly concerned that it is not getting the best quality of medical care for the dollars it spends, compared with other developed countries, as mentioned earlier. Nor has it been lost on health policy decision makers that health service researchers have questioned the depth of the scientific base on which clinical decisions presently rest in this country. Variations in physician practice styles that are difficult to explain, relating to uncertainty in medical decision making and geographic locations of medical practice, have been identified. The scarcity of valid outcome studies needed to confirm the benefits of many of the treatments and surgical procedures currently used by physicians and surgeons has also been pointed out.

Medical care has gradually become a type of mutual participatory activity in which health care decisions are believed to be a responsibility that is properly shared between physicians and patients. This view makes it even more important that physicians begin to function as patient advocates and begin to practice more as teachers of patients and less as authority figures. To be able to teach patients adequately, physicians must be able to communicate with them effectively in order to elicit their cooperation in the management of their medical problems. Unfortunately, some physicians in practice tend to believe that they are too important, or too busy, to spend much time communicating with their patients. Those physicians who continue to cling to an outmoded "doctor knows best" style of medical care should not be surprised to discover, if they take the trouble to enquire, that their practices contain a large number of dissatisfied patients.

It is not possible to give excellent medical care to patients in a quick, easy or offhand fashion, or by delegating this physician responsibility to some other professional person. Patients want and need to discuss their medical problems and concerns with their physician of choice, and they have every right to expect that this will happen. Communication nightmares for patients can be avoided by teaching all of the medical office personnel involved, including physicians, the reasons for accepting their roles as patient advocates and patient teachers, and by structuring the clinical encounter and its environment in such a way that the primary goal is not convenience for the physician, but improved outcomes of patient care from the viewpoint of patients. The overriding goal of good physician–patient communication should be to improve the outcomes of patient care from the patient's viewpoint.

There may be insensitive communication between physicians and patients for a variety of reasons, and the fault may lie with either party. Patients can be querulous, demanding, hostile, suspicious, exceedingly sensitive and highly dependent. However, a large measure of patient dissatisfaction and resentment arising from clinical encounters with physicians is due to physicians responding to these patient attitudes in a careless, thoughtless or insensitive fashion. Patting a patient's hand and saying "trust me" hardly constitutes good patient communication. Regardless of origin, insensitivity on the part of physicians can be a major deterrent to the development of effective communication with patients. Those physicians who treat patients with respect and who have recognized the need to master the techniques of good communication skills are more likely to gather full and accurate information from patients, to dispense clear and persuasive information to them and their families, and to elicit the cooperation of patients and their families with the details of suggested patient management.

Most physicians are articulate, but many nevertheless find it difficult to communicate effectively with patients. Some find it difficult to choose the appropriate level of communication for carrying out effective communication interchanges with patients because they have never learned that a less specialized level of language can be just as correct, precise and appropriate, and also can actually facilitate communication with patients and others. However, attempts by some physicians to communicate with patients and others often confuse rather than simplify the communication exchange, and the reason for this is frequently the physician's use of medical jargon, which patients very rarely fully understand. Medical jargon is a physician's conversational short cut based on the arcane terminology of the medical profession, which is rarely comprehensible to listening patients. The word "jargon" has been identified as coming from Middle English, and its original meaning was "the twittering of birds."[2] Skilled physician communicators do not need to use medical jargon, obscure medical terms or excessive medical abbreviations in their communications, because they know that their use severely limits understanding and wide dissemination of the information that is being conveyed to patients and to others.

Today's physicians, in general, are blessed with and are trained in many technical skills. Unfortunately, effective communication skills and the ability to write clearly often seem to be missing from their list of abilities. Despite the personal nature of their professional calling and a better than average educational background, physicians as a group are frequently charged with serious deficiencies in their communication and writing skills. They have been accused of filling their written material with confused thought and ambiguity, ungrammatical and pretentious written constructions, and medical jargon, and a frequent tendency to pontificate when speaking and writing. Other cited shortcomings of physician communication include a tendency to write to impress rather than to inform patients, readers or listeners, and an overuse of technical terms to the exclusion of simpler words which would help to improve the understanding of readers or listeners. Inexperienced physician writers are frequently guilty of writing sentences with subject–verb discrepancies, misplaced modifiers, and unclear or missing antecedents for pronouns.

The communication tasks that may require writing skills which physicians carry out most frequently in their professional careers, in addition to dictating office or hospital medical records, include letters to referring and other physicians, patient medical histories and physical examinations, progress notes, discharge summaries, peer-reviewed medical articles and grant proposals. Physicians who wish to learn how to write well would be best advised to keep their written words and sentences short and to the point. For example, select the word "use" over "utilize", as in the sentence "Local volunteers were used to build the playground." Long and convoluted sentences are difficult for readers to follow and are more likely to bore them than to educate them. A particular aim of good medical writing is to tell a story, to provide a word picture, to persuade a reader, or to inform a reader about a particular piece of medical information that is being presented by the physician writer.

The basic purpose of physician writing is to communicate information of importance to patients, medical colleagues and other readers, and its intrinsic value lies in the message that it conveys, the questions that it raises, and the thinking behind the decisions that it announces. In medical writing for whatever purpose, the message conveyed by the writing must always be dominant. Medical writing must satisfy the reader's need for information, not the physician writer's need for self-expression. Good physician writers understand that effective writing skills afford them a unique opportunity for learning and teaching, and for persuading others. They possess a sense of audience which directs them to write from a reader's point of view, and which enables them to keep the reader's needs for information uppermost in their mind. In the long view, better physician communication skills and enhanced patient compliance with treatment recommendations depend, in great part, on the realization by physicians that producing competent and clear prose is part of the solution. Physician writers must learn to use the correct word for each writing situation, and would do well to remember Mark Twain's words when he reminded us that "the difference between the right word and the almost right word is the difference between 'lightning' and 'lightning bug.'"

Consider this sentence from a program abstract which appeared in the printed program for a meeting of a national orthopaedic organization: "To this date, however, there have been no published studies correlating gross intra-articular anatomy and the compartments of the ankle that can be instrumented under arthroscopic visualization." The fact that there is no such verb as "instrumented" in the English language did not deter this physician author from coining a neologism. Writing and speaking are powerful and persuasive forms of medical communication, and physicians should be strongly encouraged to continually broaden and improve their skills in the techniques of both forms of communication so that they do not make such foolish mistakes in their writing efforts. It is also important for physicians to understand that each form of medical communication has different characteristics, because the written word is more formal than the spoken word. There is a need, therefore, for physicians to not only be aware of the structural and stylistic differences between spoken and written language, but also to understand and appreciate how each form of medical communication can be used most effectively. Physicians also need to think carefully about what they write in patients' charts, in consultation reports, and in medical reports of all kinds so as to get the recorded facts in the correct order in the writing effort. Careful thinking beforehand about what is to be written allows the actual writing to emerge as a more or less mechanical act.

Physician writers, because of their inherent responsibility to readers to convey clear, concise and accurate information, can best fulfill this responsibility by using precise rather than vague terms, and concrete rather than abstract words to achieve clarity of expression and meaning. Clarity of writing usually follows clarity of thought, so physician writers must first think carefully about what they want to write, and then write it as simply and clearly as possible. In medical writing, as in medical practice, being "almost right" can be dangerous and could lead to inappropriate patient outcomes. Ensuring absolute accuracy when writing is an essential element of good medical care. Good physician writing reflects the physician's ability to think logically, and physicians who learn good writing skills combine clear thinking with common language so that none of their readers will have any difficulty understanding the meaning of what has been written.

Language is the essential and perhaps the only medium by which information and ideas are transferred from one human mind to another. The first requirement of effective language is that it must be understood. The second requirement is that the information or ideas that are being transferred by the language from one person to another should not be distorted in the transfer process by factors such as faulty grammar, imprecise terms, poor word choice, disorganized sentence structure, or a writing style that is difficult to follow. The precise and accurate transfer of information by whatever means is selected is a goal that all physicians should embrace and constantly strive to achieve.

Good communication skills should be a required responsibility for physicians as professionals. Physicians need to have a clear and direct writing style, in addition to understanding exactly what they want to say, in order to be able to write clearly. In order to understand why a physician might write badly, it is necessary to look at a sentence and understand how it should work, how the ideas should be distributed through all of its different parts, and then be able to decide how to write it better. Physician writers also need to use language that is clearly understandable to readers. Impenetrable prose will impress only those physicians, patients and other readers who confuse difficulty with substance. Basically, the functions of medical writing are to tell a story, to provide a word picture, to persuade readers and to inform readers. It then becomes the obligation and responsibility of the physician writer to write clearly, without ambiguity, and with as much elegance and style as possible.

Many physicians never learned how to write clearly and effectively during their education. The very act of writing and rewriting helps physicians to clarify their ideas, to understand better what they want to say, to find the best way to organize their thoughts and their material, and to speak to the real interests and needs of their readers. The odds are poor that physicians who never learned to enjoy reading, and who have not read voraciously all their lives, will become good medical writers.[3] Physicians who wish to write must first understand what they want to say in order to be able to write it clearly and concisely. Once physicians begin to understand their own ideas better, they will start to write more clearly and will begin to understand the need both in medical writing and in medical correspondence for a clear and direct writing style. Good writing in medicine requires economy, not wordiness. It also requires physician writers to know the meanings of all the words that they choose to use, and in addition to use only words that their readers will also understand. The clear communication of ideas and concepts is the natural climax of an intellectual pursuit such as writing in medicine.

Physicians who have committed themselves to the medical profession must also be committed to providing good data to patients and others through effective communication skills. The appropriate means of communicating important information in medicine continues to be the written word. Written medical articles that are deemed worthy of being published are visible signals that the work is important and deserves to be shared with others in a report that is well written and well received. This responsibility also implies that the physician writer understands their obligations to know all of the words that they have chosen to use, and also to choose words that readers will also understand. Physicians who wish to write well also need to familiarize themselves with accepted writing techniques – for example, not beginning a new sentence with the same noun that ended the previous sentence.

Good communication skills should be a required responsibility for physicians as professionals. Physician writing styles have no set rules except for those rules set by the requirements of grammar and by a basic understanding of the English language, which offers many alternatives to physician writers. What is required for good medical writing, however, is that physicians become familiar with these alternatives. Physicians who write must consider it their responsibility to know all the words that they decide to use, and also to choose words that their readers will know. Medical writing is not a game of one-upmanship, but rather it is a game of sharing of ideas with medical readers.

Medical writing that is unclear to readers and which does not transmit a useful message to them has very little value. Physicians who wish to write in medicine must always bear in mind when beginning to write that much of the general public does not believe doctors are good communicators. Despite the personal nature of medical care and the lengthy education required, the public often perceives physicians as having serious deficiencies in their communication, writing and interpersonal skills. It is, and will remain, the responsibility of physicians to prove the public wrong because writing, speaking and communicating are skills required of all physicians. The principal purpose of this book is to assist physicians in improving their skills in these required activities of professional communication.

Chapter 2

# Good Physician Writing is a Communication Skill

The chief reason why physicians write in their professional careers is to communicate information of value to patients, colleagues and other readers, and its intrinsic value lies in the message that the writing conveys, the questions it raises, and the thinking behind the decisions that it announces. However, writing is more of an art than a science, and benefits as much from intuition as from logic. In medical writing for whatever purpose, the message conveyed by the writing must always be dominant. As mentioned in the previous chapter, medical writing must satisfy the reader's need for information, not the physician writer's need for self-expression. Consider the following sentence written by a physician in a patient's hospital medical record: "Admitted with symptoms of congestive heart failure, she requested a private room so she could be alone and undisturbed, and her family was contacted about details of her past medical history." This poor physician writer obviously had no concept of what medical information was or was not appropriate or helpful information to add to a sick patient's medical record, and as a consequence this written medical chart note was useless to this patient's future caregivers.

Physicians who write sentences like the one quoted above that contain no useful medical information about the patient's condition or prognosis have neither learned nor appreciated that words are the tools of thought. They therefore lack the ability either to write logically or to convey clearly the real message of the writing effort to readers. This failing grade in interpersonal communication should act as a warning bell to all physicians. Listening to and communicating well with patients are ancient therapeutic arts that should never be sacrificed to the severe strains associated with hospital or medical office time constraints. All too often doctors seem to lack the ability to write clearly, to speak effectively in professional settings, or to use language that patients and others can readily understand. Physicians must always remember that impenetrable prose will only impress those who confuse difficulty with substance and, for that reason, impenetrable prose must be avoided at all costs by physicians who wish to be understood by their listeners and readers. Physicians must add only pertinent patient information to hospital medical charts, and should write it so clearly that it cannot be misunderstood by any other professional person who might have cause to review a particular medical chart.

The content matter of medical communications concerns itself with critical issues such as the health and welfare of sick patients. Regardless of medical specialty or professional calling, all physicians require a common foundation of knowledge, values, professional attitudes and basic clinical skills, including the ability to communicate effectively with patients and with other physicians. Obtaining information from patients, communicating information to patients, and sharing patient information with colleagues is inherent in the practice of medicine. The fundamental rule of good physician writing is that the information being presented to readers in the writing must be so clear and complete that it can be neither misinterpreted nor misunderstood. If the physician's writing skills lack this kind of clarity, the result could be inappropriate or ineffectual patient care and even an increase in malpractice actions.

Physicians are not necessarily believed to be poor communicators at the start of their medical education, but it is thought that by the time they have completed their medical education many of them will have lost much of their communicating skills and interpersonal sensitivity. After choosing medicine as a career, physicians face additional choices concerning career options and opportunities for service. Regardless of the choices that are made, these different career paths and opportunities for service are bound together by a common thread of effective spoken and written communication. The ability to receive, record and transmit information accurately and with clarity are speaking and writing skills basic to the practice of good medicine, and these are skills that all physicians should strive to possess. However, it still needs to be emphasized to physicians that the catalysts for transforming good patient care into effective patient care are the communication and interpersonal skills of the physician providing the care. Unfortunately, all too often patients find many physicians to be deficient in these valuable clinical skills.

Experts have reported that between 55% and 70% of physician–patient communication is non-verbal. Only about 7% comprises the actual words used, and the rest consists of the physician's tone of voice, the physician's posture during patient interviews, the physician's facial expressions, and the physician's actions which suggest to the patient that the physician–patient interaction will soon be over. After a patient's successful quadruple cardiac bypass surgery, the patient's wife met the cardiac surgeon in the hospital's patient waiting area. The surgeon told the patient's wife that things went well, and predicted a rapid recovery for her husband. However, the patient's wife was very upset by the manner in which the surgeon presented his message. She later told friends that he never once looked directly at her while explaining her husband's condition, but instead looked at the walls and the ceiling during the explanation. The surgeon gave what he believed to be a clear explanation to the patient's wife, but he failed to include the recipient of his explanation in his communication effort. The non-verbal cues expressed by the surgeon's behavior suggested coldness and a lack of interest to the patient's wife, and triggered her subsequent anger.

Few physicians consider the manner in which they communicate non-verbally with patients. Non-verbal cues expressed by physicians often mirror professional attitudes and do have a positive or negative effect on patient care. Non-verbal communication can be used to communicate feelings, likings, attitudes and preferences, and tends to either reinforce or contradict feelings conveyed verbally. Good non-verbal communication by physicians is associated with patient satisfaction and understanding. The core of the physician–patient relationship is the ability of the participants to talk freely and openly with each other. Insightful and sensitive physicians have learned to interpret and respond to the nuances of both verbal and non-verbal communication exchanges between patients, their families and themselves.

Many patients also believe that doctors tend to be arrogant with patients and do not think that they do an effective job in either communicating information to them about their illness, or expressing concern to patients about their welfare. If such patient views and opinions are widespread, it is not surprising that some medical care outcomes, as viewed by patients, are less than optimal. Evidence exists that medical care, despite its professional and technical advances, may not be meeting the needs of patients, and the reason for this state of affairs is believed to be a lack of effective doctor–patient communication. Patient satisfaction with a medical experience is an important determinant of their cooperation with recommended treatment plans, and that cooperation depends more on how the physician's communication skills are perceived than on anything else. Patient satisfaction with a medical experience relates more to the doctor's communication skills than to the perceived quality of the medical care provided, the patient's waiting time, or even the cost of the medical care provided. In order to encourage patients to become better participants in their medical care and proposed treatment programs, physicians need to remember that, at best, medicine is not only a learned science but also a personal professional art. Good non-verbal communication skills reinforce the physician's verbal skills and tend to give patients a sense of connection with their physicians.

Many patients will rate their medical experience as unsatisfactory if the doctor gives them little information. Patients frequently complain that when doctors do offer explanations to them, these explanations are difficult to understand because the doctor uses obscure language and medical jargon. How well or poorly doctors communicate with their patients has a direct bearing on the accuracy of their diagnoses, and on the compliance with, satisfaction with and response to treatment of their patients. In addition, physicians must learn to appreciate economy in any written patient message, reject wordiness, and be able to choose appropriate words to use not only for their meaning but also for their value in the context of the provided message.

Physicians as a group are also widely regarded as poor writers and communicators, and the negative consequences of ineffectual writing by physicians have been a matter of concern to medical educators for some time. Many physicians live up to this unfortunate image by preferring medical jargon to clear expressions, and by sacrificing the clarity of the active voice on the altar of medical impersonality. Even worse, they are frequently blind to the imaginative side of the ideas that they work with, the so-called "big picture." The ability to write clearly and logically is recognized as an important and desirable skill for physicians to possess, but unfortunately not many physicians seem to possess this skill or even appear to try to improve their performance. Physicians can improve their writing skills once they learn to use words with the same degree of accuracy that they expect to obtain from their laboratory test results. A large part of a physician's professional responsibility is to write medical information in an office or hospital medical record of patients, and to write letters to referring physicians and others about the medical care of certain patients. Other physicians strive to write medical articles for possible publication in medical journals. Even a short experience of reviewing such communication efforts is usually sufficient to cause even the most tolerant of medical journal reviewers to wonder why so many physician writers express themselves so obscurely, so verbosely and therefore so ineffectually. Some physician writers appear to have an affinity for pompous, confusing, vague and ambiguous language. Physicians can begin to learn how to write more clearly and succinctly for readers once they start to understand that the principal purpose of their writing in medicine is to inform, not to impress.

The most frequently cited faults in material written by physicians are careless writing, confusing writing and verbose writing. The sheer awkwardness of expression exhibited by many skilled physicians when they try to write, and the ineptitude with ordinary English language revealed by other physicians, is only too commonplace. Often the cause of careless physician writing seems to be thoughtlessness on the part of the physician. Doctors who write in a careless and imprecise fashion should know better by virtue of their educational background. The following poorly composed sentence was written by a physician in the hospital medical record of a patient admitted to the hospital for a bone graft operation to correct a fracture non-union of the patient's tibia:

> There was some attempt at healing while being casted with
> some fracture callus, but the patient still had gross motion at
> the fracture site and no increase in the amount of healing on
> X-ray over the past couple of months.

Every piece of medical information that is written or dictated for appearance on a patient's hospital or medical office chart must be written so simply and clearly that there is no possibility that it could be misinterpreted or misunderstood by any future medical reader of the patient's medical record. The real danger of careless and imprecise medical writing is that it might provide careless and imprecise information about a patient's medical condition.

Despite the personal nature of their professional calling and a better than average educational background, physicians as a group are frequently charged with serious deficiencies in their writing and communication skills. Physicians have been charged with filling their written material with confused thoughts and ambiguity, an ungrammatical and pretentious writing style, medical jargon, and a frequent tendency to pontificate. Physicians frequently also exhibit tendencies to write to impress rather than to write to inform, and to use technical terms instead of simpler terms which would aid the reader's understanding. Physicians who wish to develop good writing and communication skills must first learn to avoid ambiguity, wordiness and excess words which ensure that no noun or verb goes unmodified in the writing. The ability to write well is not a natural talent for most physicians, so it will require a dedicated effort to do it well.

Physicians who wish to write well must always remember that the principal reason for writing in medicine is to inform readers, not to try to impress them. Physicians need to possess basic writing skills so that their written medical records, referral letters, and clinical and research articles are clear, concise and accurate, and convey to the reader exactly what the physician writer intended them to say, and will so appear on later retrieval and review, for whatever purpose. Medical writing is believed by many medical educators to be the most challenging, creative and rewarding of the communication skills used by physicians, mainly because of its potential for disseminating information of benefit and value both to patients and to other physicians. Developing good writing skills should be a major goal for physicians, because the nature of the medical profession is such that doctors cannot escape the need to write, be it a note on a patient's office or hospital chart, a letter to a referring physician, or an article for submission to a medical journal. Writing is a personal and sensitive skill that can be enhanced and improved to a remarkable degree by reading good writing and by writing practice.

However, for most physicians the ability to write well is not a natural talent, and therefore it takes a dedicated effort and a lot of practice to become an effective physician writer. As often as possible physician writers would be well advised to follow the writing rule that stipulates "one sentence, one idea." Putting too many details into one sentence makes it awkward and confusing for readers to follow. Consider the following sentence from a physician's dictated operative report:

> The patient was taken to the operating room and prepared and draped in the usual manner under general endotracheal anesthesia in the supine position with the knee flexed over a bolster.

In one 31-word sentence the physician who dictated this report lists five pieces of information, but leaves the reader confused and puzzled as to what actually happened to this patient. Readers of this poorly structured sentence might well wonder if the patient was prepped and draped under the anesthesia equipment, or even if the anesthetist was in the supine position.

Many physician writers seem to have difficulty in clearly expressing their thoughts and ideas about patients when writing to other physicians and to other individuals. Be it an article for possible publication, a letter to a referring physician, or a physician writer's notes on a hospital medical record, the primary reason why physicians need to write is to transfer important patient information from the mind of the transferring physician to the mind of the recipient of the written message. Good physician writing, then, must be a thoughtful process in which each word is carefully selected for use and considered both for its accuracy and for its correct placement in the sentence structure. If the physician's writing effort exhibits poor grammar, poor word choice and poor sentence structure, the writing effort will likely be ineffectual and the intended message sent by the physician will be unclear to the recipient of the message. Writing errors may be made unthinkingly by careless word choice – for example, writing "the patient's main difficulty was aortic valve disease", when medically it would be more appropriate to write "the patient's principal medical problem was aortic valve disease." Careless writing errors must also be avoided, as in the following thoughtless sentence: "A 12-man jury, half of them women, will rule on the facts."

Physicians need to possess basic writing skills so that their written records, referral letters and articles for possible publication are clear, concise and accurate, and actually say to readers exactly what the physician writer intended them to say. A tendency exists among physicians to regard medical writing as hard work and to associate all kinds of professional writing with rules and regulations of grammar and syntax, usually remembered unfavorably from earlier schooling. In truth, however, the ability to write well is recognized as an important and desirable skill for physicians to possess. Once the requisite skills have been mastered, most physicians who write well find it a liberating and enjoyable experience.

The best way to begin to learn how to become a better medical writer is to forget everything you were taught previously about writing technique. During our education, most of us were taught writing as a literary form of expression – an expressive writing form in which the writer creates a mood for the reader. However, this is the worst possible writing form to use in medical writing, because the real purpose of medical writing is to transfer information that is of value to the reader, not to create a mood for the reader. Writing was taught to most of us as one of the humanities, the literary form that emphasizes the writer's need for self-expression. If there is anything that writing in medicine does not need, it is a physician writer's self-expression. Although the more traditional education of English literature and composition may provide physicians with some knowledge of fundamental writing skills, it does not provide them with the appropriate orientation needed for writing in medicine. Confusion about the best writing form to use in medical writing has been exacerbated by college and postgraduate writing courses titled "Scientific Writing" when, of course, there is nothing at all scientific about writing. Rather, writing is a graphic form of self-expression that, although it requires familiarity with its techniques, remains a sensitive and personal skill. The question that now needs to be asked, therefore, is what is the best writing form to use for medical writing.

As mentioned previously, writing is believed by many to be the most challenging, creative and rewarding of the communication skills used by physicians because of its potential for disseminating useful information to patients and to other physicians. Clear, concise and accurate writing also has a key role in preventing medical errors at all levels of medical care. Developing good writing skills should be a major goal for all physicians, because the nature of the medical profession is such that physicians cannot escape the need to write. Writing is a personal and sensitive skill that can be enhanced to a remarkable degree by reading good writing and by writing practice. However, for most physicians the ability to write well is not a natural talent, but rather it takes a dedicated effort by the physician to become a more effective writer. Despite the personal nature of their professional calling and a better than average educational background, physicians as a group are frequently charged with serious deficiencies in their writing skills.

Often the net result for these physicians is that whatever the message they are attempting to send through their writing, it is rarely received as a fully understood message by their readers. The best way for physicians to improve both their writing skills and the lucidity of the messages that they attempt to send is to learn and use the writing form known as *technical writing*. As is true for any learned skill, attention to writing craft is what turns a collection of words into technical writing that seems natural and dynamic to readers and, in doing so, stimulates more effective medical and scientific exchanges. Physicians who understand the requirements of the language, who are able to express themselves in logically derived sentences and paragraphs, and who appreciate the roles that grammar, syntax, usage and tone play in writing will be better prepared to transfer clear and understandable information to readers by learning more about the theory and techniques of technical writing.

Chapter 3

# Technical Writing

Many physicians do not find writing a very exciting activity, and many others unfortunately find no place at all for medical writing in their professional careers. A belief exists among many physicians that professional writing is hard work, and they tend to associate it with the rules and regulations of grammar from earlier schooling. Good physician writing is indeed hard work, but only in the same sense that most worthwhile activities involve a degree of hard work. The truth of the matter is that professional writing, more than any other form of medical communication, is a creative act that can provide a unique and important kind of self-education for the physician writer, as well as bringing professional visibility and peer respect. The ability to write well is recognized as an important and desirable professional skill for physicians to possess. Good physician writing, because it is methodical and disciplined work, requires planning and organization, and the ability to translate mental images into prose. Good medical writing also requires the ability to communicate with an appropriate audience by writing in an appropriate format, followed by reading, editing and revising of what has been written.

Good style in literary writing involves many things, including having an elastic writing style so that the writing can be shaped to the writing purpose of the author. However, an elastic writing style is not appropriate for use in medical or scientific writing, because literary and medical writers have totally different purposes and reasons for writing. Thus it follows naturally that each writing form requires a different orientation toward its own writing purpose, and this orientation and writing purpose will differ significantly between these two different writing forms. Medical or scientific writing adheres to a much stricter writing form than does literary writing. In 1987, Thomas Lang, a noted American professional writer and editor, published an article in the *Journal of the American Medical Writers Association* entitled

"Medical writing is not one of the humanities."[4] His stated reason for recommending the use of this particular writing technique for medical and scientific writing was his observation over the years that his writing students and clients had very little sense of writing from the reader's point of view, and seldom anticipated or responded to the reader's need for information.

Lang believed that a different writing style was needed for medical and scientific writing so that communication with patients and others could become clearer and more effective. He noted correctly that technical writing satisfies the reader's need for information, and not the writer's need for self-expression. Technical writing, then, is the writing form that focuses on the reader's point of view and responds best to the reader's need for medical and scientific information. It is the writing form that should be used by physicians for all of their professional writing obligations and choices. The intrinsic value of technical writing lies not in what it is, but rather on what messages or pieces of information it conveys to readers, including patients. It is apparent that many medical students and physicians learned to write without any clear definitions of audience, purpose and topic, the very definitions that good technical writers use every day to guide their writing efforts.

The rules of grammar, sentence structure and syntax remain the same between these two writing styles. However, the technical writing form does require the physician writer to make precise word choices, so that there can be no opportunity for readers to misinterpret or misunderstand what has been written in the physician's message. The value of technical writing lies not in what it is, but rather in the research that it summarizes, the questions that it raises, and the thinking behind the decisions that it announces. Physicians who learn and then use the technical writing form will satisfy their readers' need for information, rather than their own need for self-expression.

Technical writing allows the physician writer to focus attention on the issues involved in communicating important medical information to readers, rather than on language issues as is frequently the case with literary writing. The primary purpose served by the technical writing format is to deliver important medical information to readers in a clear and unambiguous style by using words and sentences that, in the context of the delivered message, can be neither misunderstood nor misinterpreted by readers. Some of the characteristics of good technical writing that make it the best writing form to use for delivering medical information to readers, patients and others include its lucidity, its correctness and its completeness. The technical writing form requires physician writers to be specific in their choice of words so as to avoid reader confusion, to be accurate in the content of the material being presented to readers, and to write with such clarity that the meaning of the sentence cannot be misinterpreted.

Technical writing is now the preferred writing format for use in medicine, and is the writing style best suited to use by physician writers, because its focus is on the context of the material that is being communicated to the reader, and not on the needs and imagination of the physician writer. Good technical writing requires the physician writer to possess certain communication skills, such as a facility for the language, a familiarity with semantics, a good vocabulary, and a sense of grammar, syntax and writing structure that will allow the physician writer to convert vague thoughts into appropriate words and readable paragraphs on the page. The true value of technical writing lies not in what it is, but rather in the ease with which it communicates medical information of value to the reader. Technical and literary writing forms differ only in their orientation to the writing purpose and in their effect on the reader. Both writing forms share the same fundamental skills, such as knowledge of grammar and syntax, appropriate word choices, a sense of audience, and the ability to organize written material appropriately.

Literary writing is largely based on the free use of the writer's imagination. By contrast, the purpose of technical writing is simply to convey information of some importance and value to the physician reader in the clearest possible terms so that the reader will neither misinterpret nor misunderstand the message that is being conveyed by the written words. A physician's imagination is useful when caring for patients, but should play little role in the actual writing process and in the thoughtful thinking process that precedes the actual writing. If a piece of technical writing does not work well, the reader will have difficulty trying to understand the meaning of the written message that they are reading. Words are the precision tools that are needed to build complete understanding and effective communication in technical writing. Because the chief merit of language is its clarity, it is crucial to note at the outset that, in technical writing, the clarity of the writing will determine the effect of the written material on the reader.

The following example can serve to differentiate the style of literary writing from the style of technical writing. If asked to describe the appearance of the sky in writing, a literary writer might respond with "a solid azure blanket floats lazily overhead." This answer is full of self-expression but gives the reader little solid information about the appearance of the sky. By contrast, a technical writer would respond with "the sky is blue and cloudless", a description that can be neither misunderstood nor misinterpreted by the reader. The intrinsic value of the technical writing form relies solely on the message or piece of information that it conveys to a reader, which after all should be the principal reason why physicians write in their professional careers. Good technical writing is a combination of good word choice and good vocabulary, good sentence structure and good organization of the material, and is composed of plain, clear and simple language with the needs of the reader constantly in mind. Use of the technical writing form allows the physician writer to focus his or her attention on issues involved with communicating important medical information to the reader, rather than having to focus attention on language issues, as frequently occurs with literary writing.

The sole purpose served by technical writing is to deliver useful medical information to the reader in a clear and unambiguous style by using words and sentences that, in the context of the written text, can be neither misunderstood nor misinterpreted by the reader. Some of the characteristics of good technical writing that make it the ideal choice for use in medical writing include its lucidity, its correctness and its completeness. Technical writing is now the preferred writing format for use in medicine to deliver professional information to patients, physicians and others involved in patient care activities because, when properly written, the message that is being conveyed to readers can be neither misinterpreted nor misunderstood by them. Another requirement of good technical writing is to avoid the use of unnecessary or transitional phrases such as "interestingly" or "on the other hand", the use of "folksy" comments in the text, and the verbal expression of the physician writer's imagination unsupported by factual material.

Words are the precision tools that physician writers use to build complete understanding and effective communication when using the technical writing form, and this requirement emphasizes the need for the physician writer to understand the meaning of all words selected for use in the written material. Much of the craft of good technical writing comes from choosing words that, in the context of the written message, will mean to the reader exactly what the physician writer intended them to mean when he or she selected them. Good physician writers always try hard to find the appropriate word for the particular piece of information that they are conveying to their readers. Lack of clarity in technical writing is usually a matter of degree and most often occurs because of a careless choice of words. For example, the words "fewer" and "lesser" have frequently been used as synonyms when actually they are not synonyms at all. "Fewer" pertains to numbers, whereas "lesser" pertains to quantities. If these words are used as synonyms, the writing will lose a degree of precision, which can be a serious flaw in technical writing. Another frequent incorrect word choice among physicians is the interchangeable use of the words "patient" and "case", when in truth they are not properly interchangeable. The word "patient" is properly defined as the person with the disease or injury, and the person requiring medical care. The word "case" is properly defined as the instance or episode of disease, as in the sentence "Last year 1600 new cases of tuberculosis were reported to the US Centers for Disease Control." A quick way to remember this difference is to remind yourself that health problems come in patients, but beer and wine come in cases.

Experienced physician writers also stop and review what they have written after completing a few paragraphs, in order to make certain that their sentences are properly phrased, are grammatically correct, and say to the reader exactly what the physician writer intended them to say when writing them. Technical writing also requires the physician writer to be concise when building sentences. Do not ramble, do not overwrite, do not be verbose, and do not use two words when one would suffice. Compare the following two sentences in the context of overwriting:

> The committee discussion concerned ways to write a manual that would be useful for workers in the field (18 words).
> The committee discussed writing a field manual (7 words).

Good technical writing is a combination of good word choice and good vocabulary, good sentence structure and good organization of the material, and is composed of plain, clear language with the needs of readers constantly in mind.

When using the technical writing form, physician writers also need to develop what has been called a "sense of audience." This means that the physician writer must learn to write for the reader, not for him- or herself. A fatal mistake for physician writers who are using the technical writing format is to fall in love with their own words, which also means that they are on the wrong writing track. In addition, physician writers need to develop their writing skills so that they become adept at conveying information to readers in a form that is easily grasped and understood by them. Physician writers also must train themselves to develop a "sense of audience" by stopping the writing effort after a few paragraphs and slowly reading what has been written in order to make certain that their expressed thoughts or pieces of information are not only clearly expressed to the reader, but are also grammatically correct and do not contain unnecessary words or phrases that might dilute the meaning of the written passage. In this exercise the physician writer functions as a reader and as his or her own audience and, over time, will develop a "sense of audience" about his or her particular writing product.

Understanding and applying the following three writing concepts will help the physician writer to improve his or her technical writing skills.

1 The information in the text to be shared with readers must be written so clearly that it can be neither misunderstood nor misinterpreted by readers.
2 The physician writer must develop a "sense of audience", which means that he or she must learn to write for the reader, and not just for him- or herself.

These two concepts are put into play by frequently rereading what has been written, and by asking yourself whether what you have written is exactly what you meant to say, and whether readers will understand what you meant by the words you have chosen to present in your message. Having a sense of audience really means being able to direct the writing to the readers who will constitute the audience for the written material, and rejecting the temptation to write for the physician writer's own gratification.

3 The third concept is called "writing discrimination", which means developing a sense of content about the material, including what information, tables, graphs and illustrations to include and, equally important, what material to exclude from the manuscript.

Physicians who are good technical writers are ruthless in cutting their written material to the basic elements needed to present and support the message to readers. Periodic surveys by editors of medical journals confirm that most submitted medical manuscripts tend to be verbose and overwritten. Verbose and overwritten manuscripts are easily identified by most medical journal editors as having been written by either poor or inexperienced physician writers. A short, concise and well-written manuscript has a much greater chance of being published than a verbose and overwritten one. It should never be lost on physician writers that Watson and Crick's classic article on the chemical structure of DNA occupies only one and a half pages in a 1953 issue of *Nature*, even though it is considered to be one of the most important articles published during the twentieth century.

Medical journal editors always consider submitted manuscripts as a whole, and will review the relevance of submitted tables, graphs and illustrations with a critical eye. Medical editors will determine whether to keep or delete a particular submitted graphic on the basis of a proper appreciation of the overall value of the graphic relative to the message presented in the text. A useful general rule to follow with regard to submitted graphics is to submit no more than one table, graph or illustration per 1000 words of text. Clearly understandable figures and graphs result from careful design and from informative legends for figures, titles and footnotes for tables. Careful design of graphic material to be presented to readers is important, because figures and tables are visual means of conveying important information to them, and should therefore have a strong visual impact on the reader. Informative legends, titles and footnotes are needed to ensure that the topic of each figure and table is clear to readers. Physician writers can help themselves to develop writing discrimination by constantly asking themselves as they write "Is this piece of information or this graph, table or illustration absolutely essential to the accurate and complete coverage of my topic?" If the answer is no, as it often will be, the material in question should be deleted. If the physician writer has built their story to a logical climax and has stated their ideas clearly and forcefully, readers will grasp the ideas and conclusions offered in the article. Always remember that authors in general are more concerned with content, whereas editors and manuscript reviewers are more concerned with its expression.

Above all else, physician writers must reject the temptation to fall in love with their own material and with their selected words or phrases. If this should happen, it means that the physician writer has not yet learned the rules of successful technical writing. The first rule that underlies successful technical writing in medicine is always to write for the reader in completely understandable words, phrases and sentences. The second rule of good technical writing in medicine is for the physician writer to understand that they are simply the messenger who is providing useful medical information of value to medical readers, and that they are definitely neither a storyteller nor an entertainer. Unlike spelling, which need not be perfect because software programs now check spelling and offer alternative words, a sentence that is grammatically unclear or badly written stands out like an uninvited guest at a fancy dinner party.

Good technical writing in medicine is a combination of good data, good vocabulary, good sentence structure and good organization of the material, and is written in plain and clear language with the needs of readers constantly in mind. Good data is the physician writer's responsibility as the reporting author, and derives from the research performed and the data collected by the author(s) for the planned article. Good vocabulary pertains to correct word choice in the writing, and can be best achieved by being an avid reader, as this familiarizes physician writers with multiple word choices, their meanings, and their appropriate placement and use in a medical article. A good vocabulary goes hand in hand with a love of reading. Good sentence structure means constructing sentences that are grammatically correct and which place the main point or main idea of the sentence at the beginning of the sentence. To some degree, good sentence structure also bears a relationship to the use of the active or passive voice in the writing. If the subject of the sentence performs the action (for example, "John caught the ball"), the verb is in the active voice. If the subject of the sentence receives the action of the sentence (for example, "the ball was caught by John"), the verb is in the passive voice. Most medical journal editors would prefer physician writers to use the active voice more frequently because they want each sentence to carry its own weight, and because the active voice tells readers who did what to whom. Unfortunately, a lot of published medical writing makes for dull reading because it tends to be written in the passive voice.

Three guiding principles should be followed by physician writers when using the technical writing format for their medical articles and communications.

1  A principal rule of good technical writing is to write with a "sense of audience." This means being constantly aware during the construction of the text that what you are doing as a medical writer is simply transferring information from your mind to the mind of the reader, so as to stay on track during the writing process.
2  As much as possible use simple and easily understood language in the writing, and studiously avoid using medical jargon which, more often than not, will be out of place and will only confuse readers who are not familiar with the particular jargon used.

3 Write the text in the technical writing format and do it so clearly that it becomes impossible for readers to misinterpret or misunderstand what has been written. A mistakenly placed modifier, for example, can destroy the sense of a written sentence, as in the following example: "Abraham Lincoln wrote the Gettysburg Address on the trip from Washington on the back of an envelope."

The precise and accurate transfer of information by the written word is a goal that all physician writers should embrace and constantly strive to achieve, because it is the essence of good technical writing in medicine, and is the most effective way for physician writers to transfer useful medical information to other physicians and other readers. The best way for physician writers to achieve this goal in their writing efforts is to use the technical writing format whenever they have occasion to write in their professional duties and obligations.

Chapter 4

# Preparing to Write

It must be assumed that physicians who wish to write for the medical literature are already familiar with examples and exercises involving such important writing details as parallel construction, agreement of subject and verb, references of pronouns, dangling, trailing and misplaced modifiers, and other grammatical obligations. Many inexperienced physician writers do not know how the language works – for example, why certain constructions are allowed and others are not. As a result, their writing attempts may contain subject–verb disagreements, misplaced modifiers, and unclear or missing antecedents for pronouns.[5] Before beginning the work of collecting data and information about a proposed study that a physician wishes to write about and submit to a medical journal for possible publication, the physician writer would be well advised to give some thought to which journal might be best suited to publish the paper when it has been written. Physician writers also need to appreciate from the start of the writing effort that the manuscript acceptance rate for unsolicited articles in this country ranges from a high of 64% (*Mayo Clinic Proceedings*) to a low of 7% (*New England Journal of Medicine*).[6] The best advice for most physician writers is to submit their finished article to the journal that seems most appropriate to the strength of the submitted article and to reader interest in the topic.

The prospective physician author should also carefully review the Information for Authors section in the journals that he or she is considering for the editorial review of the planned manuscript. This section tells the physician writer about the editorial interests of the particular journal, what types of medical manuscripts the journal prefers to consider for publication, and usually offers some general information about the editorial requirements of the particular journal. Information is also usually provided about manuscript preparation, preferred writing style and length, and preferred reference style. Most medical journals publish this information in at least two issues per year under a heading such as "Information for Authors."

Ranking as equal in importance with the content matter of the written material is the need for readers of the published journal article to be able to clearly understand what has been written in the article. Medical writing, like all science writing, is persuasive writing and it must be based on fact and logic, not on supposition or speculation. Whether or not the physician writer achieves this goal will largely depend on the words chosen for use in the written material. The writing of a critically reviewed and accepted journal manuscript will be found to be characterized by writing cleanliness, accuracy in reporting the factual material, and brevity in the use of the English language. Above all, prospective medical authors must learn to omit needless and superfluous words from the written text. Style in medical writing has no set rules because the English language offers many alternatives from which to choose. Good medical writing involves many things, including being flexible so that the writing can be shaped to the physician writer's purpose. Physician writers can retain their own particular writing style so long as it follows the general guidelines adopted for medical writing by medical journals.

Two key elements required for organizing the writing effort successfully and efficiently are a thorough literature search before beginning the writing effort, and the use of an outlining technique to organize the collected material for the actual writing effort. A thorough literature search at the beginning of the writing effort can tell the physician writer if the same or similar material has been reported or published before, and will frequently provide additional avenues of investigation for the physician writer to consider. An effective medical writing style begins with a clear sense of purpose and with an outlining scheme of some kind to group together bits of information or data collected previously in the physician writer's notes. Outlining is the organizational scheme that lies at the heart of the traditional approach to medical writing for publication, particularly for those physicians who have not yet written much material for publication. Outlining also serves as an excellent device to allow physician writers to gain control of complex ideas, and allows them to slot these ideas into their proper niches in the writing effort.

An outline is a tool that is used by the physician writer mainly for the benefit of the reader. The perception of relationships between data helps to focus the physician writer's literature search and can be the key to organizing the writing effort. Clear organization of the collected material into appropriate subdivisions of the whole effort leads to clear thinking and writing, and is the principal reason why experienced physician writers make use of an outlining technique as a writing blueprint at the start of the writing process. Structure, the architectural dimension of technical writing, is best applied to the writing by beginning the writing effort by constructing a temporary manuscript outline. The longer the piece of writing, the greater is the need for a preliminary writing outline. An outline is not an art form, nor is it meant to be read by a reader. It is simply a tool that physician writers can use for the benefit of physician readers who are conditioned to appreciate a neat and logical development of ideas.

Theoretically, a good outline design should lead to an interesting piece of writing because, without a preliminary outline, the structure and substance of the medical writing may lead to a finished product that appears to many readers to be disorganized. To avoid dullness in reading, the physician's writing must be substantive, interesting and even graceful, and the physician writer must understand at the onset that outlining does not necessarily contribute anything to those qualities. What outlining does contribute is a neat and orderly way to arrange the facts and ideas to be reported in the completed article. Because outlining is a means rather than an end, it may not be necessary for more experienced physician writers. However, the longer the planned piece of writing, the greater is the need for the use of an outline for the design of the planned medical article. Structure is the architectural dimension of medical writing, and nothing helps reader comprehension more than the clear and logical march of ideas. Outlining is the best method currently available for achieving such structure. Good organization of a manuscript allows readers and editorial reviewers to concentrate on the presented material without being distracted by a poor writing structure. Outlining is simply a technique used by physician writers to gather their thoughts and their collected information about the topic under consideration into some kind of logical sequence or structure. Outlining addresses organization, and organization results in a more logical development of the written material and, in the long run, a better final product.

Although outlining is useful in a physician's writing efforts, its primary purpose is to function as a blueprint method for planning the writing of medical articles and research reports. Available outlining techniques allow physician writers to focus separately on small segments of information, so they can be concerned with only one kind of organizational structure at a time. The advantage of this type of focus is that it helps physician writers to balance the emphasis that needs to be given to each part of the writing plan. Regardless of which type of outlining technique is chosen by the physician writer, outlining should not be overly detailed but should simply be used as a tool for organizing both the material and other ideas to help them to structure their ideas and concepts by acting as a scaffolding at the start of the writing process. Informal outlines are less structured and are better suited to the purposes of physician writers than are the more structured outlines usually taught in English composition classes.

Three types of informal outlining techniques that are useful for medical writing are listed below.

1  *Mind mapping* or the *spoke wheel technique*. Mind mapping, a technique designed to stimulate a free flow of ideas, is the brainstorming that a physician writer performs with him- or herself before starting the actual writing process. The writer begins by writing the theme or main topic of the proposed article on a sheet of paper and then enclosing it in a circle. He or she then encloses other main and subordinate points as they come to mind, and connects the circles with branch lines. One advantage of this type of free flow idea outline is that it reveals relationships between ideas and data without forcing the ideas and data into a formal structure. These relationships can be changed by the writer as the map develops and other relationships become apparent. This informal outlining technique can be rearranged as necessary to suit the logic of the main points developed by the outlining process. Mind mapping is a personal outlining technique, and the relationships developed by the map are those determined by the physician writer.

2  *Idea (issue) tree technique*. When completed, the interrelationships developed by this technique bear a resemblance to a Christmas tree on the paper. When using this technique the physician writer arranges ideas, data and other pieces of information in hierarchical order by deciding what pieces of information to include or exclude, by deciding how these pieces of information fit together or are related, and by constructing the tree with the main topics at the top of the tree and related issues and topics branching out from it and from one another according to their importance and relationship to each other and to other ideas.

3  *IMRAD format*. IMRAD is an acronym for the most frequently used outlining technique for the organization and writing of articles for

publication in the medical literature. This acronym stands for Introduction, Materials and Methods, Results and Discussion, which represent the sections or subdivisions that make up the preferred structure for articles submitted for publication in the medical literature. More specific details relating to this format are given in Chapter 5. Physician writers can also use the IMRAD format as an outlining technique because it is convenient and simple to use, but it may require frequent revisions as the writing ideas develop and come to the physician writer's mind. For example, an idea that was originally placed in the Introduction section may later be seen to fit better in the Discussion section, after all the pieces of evidence have undergone final review by the physician author.

Because outlines are only informal aids to structuring the written information, physician writers should never hesitate to alter their outlines as they develop, and as the accumulating information suggests or indicates to the physician writer. Writing outlines are usually discarded after they have served their purpose in the writing effort because their sole purpose is to help physician writers to develop and arrange their material appropriately before starting to write their planned article.

## An Overview of the Process of Writing and Getting Published

1 *Thinking.* Plan the text around the topic, purpose and audience.
   - What is your topic of interest?
   - What type of information do you have to contribute to this topic?
   - What readership do you wish to address?
   - Develop the major idea for the study or project.
   - Write notes as ideas and suggestions for additional topics come to mind and are developed more fully.
   - Think carefully about what needs to be said and focus on the points that need to be presented by writing notes to yourself as the focusing progresses.
2 *Planning.*
   - Plan or organize the material and its development by using an outlining technique. Outlining is based on the premise that research and thinking should precede the actual writing process.

- Gradually develop the form of the idea and the points to be presented in the article or written material.
- Refine the developed ideas and points so as to focus on essential data, and exclude material that is irrelevant, redundant or speculative with regard to the purpose of the written material.

3 *Physician writer's file.* Many physician writers find it helpful at the beginning of the writing process to create and maintain a binder or file containing the following:

- notes detailing the physician writer's thoughts and decisions pertaining to the proposed article's direction and content
- the physician writer's outlining notes
- a copy of each article that the physician writer plans to reference and use in his or her completed text
- a photocopy of the Instructions for Authors section from a selected journal
- a copy of a recent article from a targeted journal so that the physician writer can become familiar with the journal's writing style.

## Sentences

In medical writing it is best to present the main point or main idea of a sentence at the beginning of the sentence so that readers can begin with a clear idea of where the physician writer is going with the information.

For example, ''The mosquito was identified as the carrier of yellow fever by Carlos Finlay, an 1855 graduate of Jefferson Medical College'' is much clearer than ''Carlos Finlay, an 1855 graduate of Jefferson Medical College, is credited with identifying the mosquito as the carrier of yellow fever.''

Good physician writers constantly read over previously written sentences and paragraphs to guard against careless writing errors, which unfortunately may occur quite frequently. A modifier, word, phrase or clause that is incorrectly placed next to a word that it does not sensibly describe is said to be a misplaced or dangling modifier, as in the following example:

> The patient left the operating room in good condition (incorrect placement).
> The patient was in good condition on leaving the operating room (correct placement).

It is the condition of the patient that the physician should be concerned about, not the condition of the operating room.

Correct word choice for a particular writing situation will depend largely on the physician writer's depth of vocabulary and knowledge of word meaning. Lack of clarity in medical writing is frequently a matter of degree that arises from a careless choice of words. Physician writers should always resolve word usage questions in the direction of greater precision and clarity in the sentence in question. Frequent reference to a dictionary or a thesaurus will help to expand the physician writer's range of vocabulary and knowledge of word meaning. A good vocabulary and a broad understanding of word meaning allow a choice of words that will be accurate for the occasion, and which will fit well in the context in which the words are being used. Much of the craft of medical writing lies in choosing words that, in the context of the text, will mean to the reader exactly what the physician writer intended them to mean. Good physician writers try hard to find the appropriate word for particular writing situations, because no word is in itself good or bad, or right or wrong. Whether a particular word is accurate or not in the context in which it is being used will depend greatly on the physician writer's depth of vocabulary and knowledge of word meaning. A good vocabulary and a broad understanding of word meanings allow a choice of words that will be accurate for the particular writing situation, and which will fit well in the context in which the words are being used. Physician writers should try hard to find the appropriate words for each particular writing situation. Whether a particular chosen word is accurate or not in the context in which it is being used, or whether or not it is put to good use in the writing effort, can only be judged in the context of the writing situation and the message that is being sent to readers. At all times, physician writers should strive to reflect clarity and grace in their written messages, in addition to the necessary medical details.[7]

When the physician writer is ready to begin writing their text, they should organize the writing effort around the following four basic instructions for good medical writing.

1  Clarity – which means not trying to make each sentence in the writing do too many things. Be guided by the rule of restriction, which advises one idea per sentence. Construct paragraphs with simple declarative sentences that follow each other in logical sequences. Use plain ordinary words, even one-syllable words when possible, to get the message across to readers.

2 Simplicity – which means getting rid of word clutter, pompous frills in the writing, verbal bloating, and the use of needless and repetitive qualifiers.

3 Economy – which means in medical writing that short is better than long. Use plain good English, avoid unnecessary medical jargon and fancy buzzwords, and make the writing crisp and lean. Always keep in mind during the writing process that medical journal editors have long maintained that most submitted manuscripts are verbose and grossly overwritten.

4 Humanity – which means never say anything in the writing that you would not be comfortable saying in conversation with other physicians. This can also be called a writer's choice of words. Always remember that much of the craft of medical writing comes from choosing words that, in the context of the text, will mean to readers exactly what the physician writer intended them to mean when written. Unfortunately, too many physician writers have a tendency to choose complicated and unusual words when simpler words would be preferable for better reader comprehension.

After the physician writer has organized their material by using an outlining technique, they can begin to plan the structure of the written article.

1 Develop and refine the major topic for the article or project. Write notes to yourself as ideas and suggestions for additional topics or subtopics come to mind and are developed more completely.

2 Think carefully about what needs to be said, and focus on the points that need to be presented in the finished article.

3 Search the pertinent literature thoroughly for relevant background information and to make certain that the proposed study, or a similar study, has not been published previously.

4 Plan or organize the development of the article by using an outlining technique.

5 Gradually develop the form of the idea for the article, and its supporting data, for presentation in the article.

6 Write according to the format recommended by the selected journal to which you plan to submit the completed manuscript.

7 Begin to arrange the collected data and material under the four main headings of Introduction, Materials and Methods, Results and Discussion.

Writing a competent medical article with a good chance of publication is largely dependent upon following these basic instructions.

1 Think logically during the planning and organization of the material. Clear medical writing follows clear thinking, which follows the use of an effective outlining technique.
2 Analyze the data or evidence rigorously and interpret it critically.
3 Organize the relevant material in a clearly understood and lucid fashion before starting to write. The headings of Introduction, Materials and Methods, Results and Discussion can also be used in this organizational effort.
4 Present the results of the study in clearly understood text and in the appropriate writing format.
5 The final result of the writing effort should be presented to readers in a clear and concise fashion, but at the same time should be pleasing to read.
6 In its final form, the finished article should be of a length just sufficient to present the results obtained to the reader clearly and succinctly. The final form of the manuscript must be free of bloated text and extraneous pieces of information that the author has used merely for extra padding. Reviewing past copies of the journal to which the author plans to send the manuscript will give a clear indication of the proposed journal's preferred word count.

Exercising "due diligence" in medical writing requires the physician writer to adopt the following approach.

1 Take a reader-centered approach to medical writing. Keep readers and their needs constantly in mind.
2 Stress "readability" in the article during preparation and writing.
3 Weigh each written word carefully for appropriateness and accuracy. Always choose the most appropriate word or phrase for each writing circumstance.
4 Be certain that every sentence means to the reader exactly what the physician writer intended it to mean when he or she wrote it. For example, do not write "The 20 excluded patients are displayed in Table 2", but rather write "The 20 patients who were excluded from the study are listed in Table 2."

Standard writing formats are used in medical and scientific writing because medical and scientific prose is difficult in itself, and a standardized writing format, which breaks the material down into distinctive parts, makes it easier for both physician writers and their readers to know exactly how the material in the article will be presented. After all the data have been collected, analyzed and thoroughly understood by the physician writer, the writing itself often emerges as a relatively mechanical act, requiring of the physician writer only a reasonable command of basic English sentence structure.

Chapter 5

# Writing for Publication

Physician writers who wish to have their written material published must strive to learn and use a prose style that is lean, clear, accurate, concise and completely free from medical jargon. Professional jargon has no place in good medical writing because its use limits understanding of the message to those few readers who are familiar with the particular jargon used. Physician writers can maintain their own writing styles so long as the meaning of their written material is accurately and effectively conveyed to the reader. Just as listening to and communicating with patients is an essential part of good patient care, using clear and uncomplicated language in the construction of medical text is an essential part of good physician writing. Physicians who wish to write for publication in the medical literature should attach to their writing efforts the same degree of importance that they attach to physician–patient communication and to physician–patient relationships. Physician writers must understand that common words are learned faster and remembered longer than uncommon words, and for that reason must strive not to use obscure medical language and medical jargon in the construction of their medical texts.

The purpose of structure in medical writing is to allow the transfer of important information and meaning from the mind of a physician writer to the mind of a reader in a clear and precise fashion. Structure in medical writing makes the offered information easier for readers to grasp, understand and remember. Structural problems that are frequently encountered in material written by physicians can include errors in grammar, faulty punctuation and poor sentence structure. Important points made in publishable medical articles should be delivered to readers in carefully constructed paragraphs, which are important pieces of medical writing structure.[8]

Paragraphs are the writing structures in which relevant facts or ideas are presented to readers, and in which facts and ideas that have already been presented are developed for better reader understanding. Paragraphs are composed of groups of related statements presented as units to readers by the physician writer. Each sentence in a paragraph is a unit of the fact or idea being presented to the reader, or a step in contributing to the construction of the idea or concept. The lead sentence in a paragraph should be clear and direct, with the main point of the sentence leading off, as in the following sentence:

> The number of African-American physicians in the USA must be increased to provide adequate health care to meet the projected increases in the minority populations in the years ahead.

A paragraph begins with a topic sentence and moves on to the supporting details. However, the whole paragraph should be able to stand alone as a unit of a complete idea. Sentences supplying small pieces of information to the development of the idea that is being presented to readers should be connected together smoothly to form the paragraph, which is the writing form that physician writers need to depend upon to present their material and their ideas to readers. The trick of writing a good paragraph for a medical article is to find the right fit in the manuscript between the given format and each element of style, including vocabulary, content, writing tone, sentence structure and paragraphs and the overall written manuscript.

Physician writers must understand that they need to become masters of paragraphs because sentences in the text must be put together into a block, and it is that block of words that governs the ideas in and determines the direction of good writing in the construction of medical articles for publication. Paragraphs are not ends in themselves, but rather they are parts of a larger structure. What they are not, and should never become, are random accumulations of written sentences. Whenever possible, each paragraph should lead with a topic sentence that serves to alert readers to the facts and ideas that will follow. A paragraph functions as an important structural unit of the writing because of the connections that should exist between the statements contained in the paragraph. Each paragraph should contain at least four sentences, and should appear as a unit to readers because it is structurally set off from what precedes it and from what follows it, either by indentations or by spacing above and below it. Sentences written in English are clearest, most forceful and easiest to understand if they are simple and direct in their construction. If complicated and indirect sentences tend to dominate a paragraph in a medical article, difficulty will be created for readers, and the physician writer's message will risk being unclear to readers. Paragraphs may also end with a statement of summation if this is desired by the physician writer.[9]

Before beginning the writing effort, the physician writer should read Chapter 3 on technical writing again, and also give some thought to which of the many medical journals available might be most receptive to the finished and submitted manuscript. Medical journals vary widely in their fields of interest and subject matter, and the physician writer would be well advised to give some thought to trying to match the finished text and its subject matter to the self-described interests and goals of particular medical journals. The aim of this effort is to try to select a medical journal whose publishing goals fit well with the subject matter to be presented by the physician writer(s) in the completed manuscript. Prospective physician authors will also find it profitable to visit medical libraries to familiarize themselves with the kinds of articles that are published in particular medical journals.

Published medical articles are still the principal method used for the wide exchange of medical information. A published medical article lists other medical and scientific literature information relative to the problem being studied and reported, provides sufficient description of the methodology used to enable the study to be repeated by others if desired, allows for a comprehensive discussion of the results and, most importantly, can be subjected to a process of peer review before it is accepted or rejected for publication. Medical journals differ widely in subject matter published, style, degree of specialization, frequency of publication, circulation and readership, editorial policy and prestige. Some medical journals are highly specialized, while others are more general with regard to scope of published material. It is important for physician writers to learn to target their articles to appropriate medical journals.

Physician writers must also understand that the editorial rejection rate for articles submitted to some peer-reviewed journals can run as high as 80%. Reasons for rejection might include manuscripts that are considered inappropriate for that particular journal, articles that are not considered original enough to warrant publication, manuscripts that contain gross inaccuracies or claims by the author(s) that are not supported by the data presented, and manuscripts that are too long or that are presented so poorly that no amount of revising or copy editing will correct the identified problem. Even if the article presents the author's own analysis and findings, it might still duplicate material published previously in the same or another journal. However, if the presented data or evidence opens up an entirely new approach to a previously well-covered subject, the article should stand a good chance of being accepted for publication. What is required for successful medical publication is a good idea or concept backed up by a good study design, good data to support the conclusions, and the ability of the physician writer to organize and present the material concisely and in such a way that it is both understandable and interesting to medical journal readers, and is within the journal's preferred word length. However, the key individuals who need to be convinced of the worthiness of the submitted manuscript are the medical journal editor and his or her selected manuscript reviewers.

Journal editors will acknowledge receipt of the submitted manuscript, and will usually estimate approximately how much time they will require for the evaluation. Assuming that the author(s) have submitted a well-thought-out and well-written manuscript to an appropriate medical journal, they can rely on the journal editor to arrange for a fair reading and evaluation of the submitted manuscript. The selected professional editorial reviewers of the submitted manuscript are, and will remain, unknown to the submitting author(s). However, the author(s) of the submitted article must learn to detach their egos from the writing and reviewing process, and wait for the journal's response with patience. Editors and manuscript reviewers often report that many authors who submit manuscripts to them for editorial review do not adhere to the journal's format and editorial policies, which tends to start the submission process off on the wrong foot. Submitting medical authors must be certain that the length of their manuscripts is close to the target journal's average length requirement, and ideally it should be a bit shorter. The number of submitted tables, graphs, figures and references should also be close to the journal's stated average. Physician writers must learn to use short sentences and short paragraphs, because the best medical articles tend to be concise. Some journals measure article length by word count. For example, the *New England Journal of Medicine* requires manuscripts to be less than 3000 words, while the *British Medical Journal* limits original text to no more than 2000 words, with a maximum of six tables or illustrations.[10]

# Constructing the Text for Medical Articles

Each component of the completed manuscript should begin on a separate page in the following sequence.

1  Title.
2  Abstract and key words.
3  Text.
4  Acknowledgments (if any).
5  References.
6  Tables and figures. Each table and figure, complete with titles and footnotes, must be on a separate text page.
7  Legends for illustrations.

# Title of the Medical Article

The title of a written medical article, which is always placed on the first page of the manuscript, is a label used to identify the contents of the article to readers, and should be carefully chosen because it may be selected for inclusion in an abstract, the *Index Medicus* or an online database. The selected title should serve to identify the main topic of the article and to attract the attention of potential readers. Good titles are simple, short and concise, and should contain an accurate promise of the article's content, all within a reasonable word length. The title should be expressed in the fewest words possible that adequately describe the article's content or thrust, but must also serve to pique the interest of readers, and to classify or identify the article for indexing and abstracting services. An uninformative title carries the risk of deterring or misleading readers. Often a title is not a sentence, nor does it have to be. However, the order in which the title words are presented to readers is important. All of the words in the title must be chosen carefully and their association with one another managed thoughtfully. The most frequently encountered errors in defective titles, and the most damaging in terms of reader comprehension, are inappropriate word choice and faulty syntax or word order.

The words that are used in the title should be limited to those that highlight the significant content of the article in terms that are both meaningful to the reader and retrievable in bibliographic searches. The title, along with the names of the author and co-authors and the names of their respective institutions, should always appear on the title page or first page of the manuscript. The title page should also include the name of the sponsoring department and institution to which the work should be attributed, as well as the name and address of the particular author selected to be the corresponding author, along with his or her email address. If the selected title of the manuscript does not capture the attention of readers, the Introduction section of the published paper must do so.

## The Abstract

Abstracts are summaries of completed articles and, depending upon the type and purpose of the abstract, they are written in a certain prescribed form, in a certain number of words and in the past tense. Abstracts help readers to select appropriate articles quickly and allow for more precise literature searches. Because abstracts are a way for readers to preview published articles, the abstract needs to be as clear and direct as possible while at the same time touching on all the important points made in the published article, and it must do so within a short prescribed word count. A good abstract helps to attract reader attention to the published article. The selected journal's preferred abstract word count will be found in the journal's Instructions for Authors section in previously published issues of the selected journal.

For far too many physician writers, the abstract is the last piece of information to be written during the preparation of the manuscript, often just before the completed manuscript is sent to a medical journal for editorial review. Many physician writers tend to give little thought to writing the abstract in their hurry to finish the manuscript and send it off which, unfortunately for them, may prove to be a great mistake. Journal editors have a habit of periodically checking the accuracy of submitted abstracts against the data contained in the manuscript. It could be embarrassing for a physician writer to have their manuscript rejected by the journal because the information in the submitted abstract bears little or no resemblance to the material in the submitted manuscript. This may happen if the abstract is written as an afterthought rather than as an integral part of the submitted manuscript. Good abstract writing takes practice, but physician writers will find this practice to be a worthwhile effort, and will soon begin to understand why an abstract should not only be well written, but also be written earlier rather than later in the development of the article.

An informative (comprehensive) abstract is the type of abstract often found in published medical articles. This form of abstract briefly describes the content material of the article, and is constructed from information contained in the Introduction, Materials and Methods, Results and Discussion sections of the article. An informative abstract provides an overview of the findings reported in the published article, and should serve to stimulate reader interest in the publication. The abstract, as a short summary of the published article's major arguments, findings and conclusions, can be constructed by responding to the following statements.

- This is what we studied.
- This is how we did it.
- This is what we learned.
- This is what we believe the findings mean.

Abstracts have a predetermined word count, which can be found in the Instructions for Authors section of the selected journal, and are thus limited to a short description of the problem investigated in the study and its solution as proposed by the author(s). When constructing an abstract, the following organizational outline should be used.

1 A topic sentence that gives readers some information about the background of the problem investigated and the reason(s) for performing the study.
2 A brief description of the methods used in the study.
3 A summary of the observed results.
4 A conclusion summarized from the Discussion section of the article, which gives the reader a sense of relationship to the topic that led off the abstract.

A different type of abstract, called a structural abstract, has been used by many peer-reviewed journals since 1991. This abstract is fashioned on the belief that structure should replace the fluid but often uninformative prose of more traditional abstracts. Structure in this type of abstract ensures that the essential elements of an organized study, such as objective, design, setting, patients, outcome measures, results and conclusions, are provided in a more consistent and complete manner for readers, reviewers and those searching databases. A structural abstract ensures that the reader knows what research questions were asked, what was measured and what was found. Structural abstracts for original studies require authors to systematically disclose the objective, the basic research design, the clinical setting, the participants, the interventions (if any), the main outcome measurements, the results and the conclusions. This abstract design provides the key information needed by readers for selecting articles of relevance and quality for their own reading. This style of abstract writing is, for example, now standard for all articles published in the *Journal of the American Medical Association*, among other major medical journals.

A structural abstract for an original medical article contains the following headings.

1 Objective: the exact question(s) addressed by the article.
2 Design: the basic study design.
3 Setting: the location and level of clinical care.
4 Patients or participants: the manner of selection and the number of patients or participants who entered and completed the study.
5 Interventions: the exact treatment or intervention, if any.
6 Main outcome measures: the primary study outcomes as planned before data collection began.
7 Results: the key findings.
8 Conclusions: major conclusions including direct clinical applications. The content of Conclusions provides a brief summary of the importance of the research question asked or the clinical question examined, enables the reader to determine how the study results and conclusions advance the field, and defines their implications for clinical medicine or for medical research.

## The Organization of Medical Manuscripts

When reading published medical articles, one is struck by a certain amount of 'sameness' about them. This sameness relates to the form or structure of the published article, not to its contents, and originates from the fact that published medical articles are deliberately organized in a similar fashion so that medical readers can concentrate on the medical facts contained in the published medical article. This organizational format is known as IMRAD, an acronym that stands for Introduction, Materials and Methods, Results and Discussion as they relate to the structure of the written article. This type of published orientation, although not very exciting in print, is deliberate in intent so that all medical articles will appear in a similar published format, thereby allowing a clearer understanding of the presented purpose and result of a particular medical article.

## Introduction

This section deals with two questions.

1  What is the problem being studied?
2  What is the question that needs answering?

The Introduction, which is written in the present tense, presents the purpose and scope of the article to readers, provides the background information needed by readers to fully understand the study, may vary in length from a few sentences to several pages, and should make the topic of the article seem interesting or important to readers. The main purpose of the Introduction is to tell readers why the study was conducted, and what gaps in the knowledge base the author(s) believe needed to be filled. The Introduction should supply sufficient background information to allow readers and editorial reviewers to understand and evaluate the results of the reported study without having to refer to previous publications on the same or similar subjects. Few references should be cited in the Introduction, but they must be selected carefully to provide only the most important and relevant information to readers and reviewers.

The steps involved in writing an Introduction can be summarized as follows.

1  Present the nature and scope of the problem being investigated in clear language and in the present tense. Tell the reader why the problem investigated in the study was considered significant enough by the author(s) to be examined further.
2  Review the pertinent literature selectively, and include only the most relevant studies for the reader to refer to in order to orient them to the direction taken by the study.
3  Tell the reader the method of investigation selected and, if necessary, the author's reasons for selecting this particular method of investigation.
4  State the principal results obtained in the study or investigation.
5  Conclude the Introduction with a specific statement of purpose, such as "The purpose of this investigation was to report the results obtained when drug X was used for the first time in the treatment of 100 consecutive children with whooping cough."

## Materials and Methods

This section describes how the problem was solved, or how the question was answered. Written in the past tense, the Materials and Methods section must contain full and specific details of the investigative method used in the reported study, because a major purpose of this section is to provide readers and editorial reviewers with enough specifics and details of the investigative method that was used to allow other competent workers in the same field to repeat the same research if they wish to do so. Scientific validity demands very careful writing of this section of the manuscript, because the cornerstone of the scientific method requires that the methods used and the results obtained in the study be reported in full and sufficient detail and in a form that would allow others to reproduce the same results, if desired, in order to be judged of scientific merit by other investigators in the same field. For this reason, medical journal editors and manuscript reviewers require physician writers to be precise about the details of the study and the investigative methods used when describing these items in the Materials and Methods section. If required due to the nature of the study, prior approval for the study must be obtained from the Institutional Review Board (IRB) of the principal author's institution.

The Materials and Methods section must address the following points.

1  After the hypothesis underlying the study has been noted, the selected study design is described in full and precise detail. The hypothesis under study is usually not repeated here in basic scientific articles, but rather it is stated in the Introduction.
2  Subjects (patients, animals, etc.) to be studied must be defined and characterized as fully as possible in order to minimize variations caused by uncontrollable variables. The selected journal may require the author(s) to submit a statement that the Institutional Review Board of the senior author's institution has given permission to the author(s) for human subjects to be studied.
3  Interventions used in the study (surgical procedures, treatments, drugs, etc.) must be described in detail. The use of controls and other measures to minimize bias must be explained.
4  Measurements, methods and other relevant observations must be described fully.
5  Statistical methods used to assess the observed data must be described fully.
6  If animals have been used in the study, the selected journal may

require assurance from the author(s) that the protocols for the animal studies have been approved by the Institutional Animal Care and Use Committee of the senior author's institution.

## Results

This section describes what was found by doing the study. Written in the past tense, the Results section is crucial to the structure of the article because it presents to the readers of the published article the new information learned by the author(s) as a result of doing the study. The Introduction told readers what problem or question was studied and why. The Materials and Methods section told readers how the problem was solved or how the posed question was answered. The Results section tells readers what results were obtained by doing the reported study. Because of its critical importance to the total writing effort, the Results section must be written clearly without verbiage and, most importantly, it must be written so that the results obtained in the study are able to speak for themselves without any unnecessary embellishment by the author(s). Physician writers must take particular care not to overwrite the Results section, but rather let the results of the study and the information obtained by doing the study speak for themselves.

The purpose of the Results section is to tell readers and reviewers what the study design, described previously in the Materials and Methods section, was able to accomplish or discover during the study period. The following points should be borne in mind when writing the Results section.

1 The physician writer should first provide an overall description of the study or research, thus providing the reader with the "big picture" without having to repeat the study details already given in the Materials and Methods section.
2 Only summarized or representative data derived from the study results need to be presented. Physician writers must avoid presenting data in endlessly repetitive detail, because this will only bore readers. Numerical data can usually be presented in tables or graphs. If the data are set up in a table, the text only needs to point out what differences in the data were found, or call attention to a lack of statistically significant correlations in the presented data. Graphics is a generic term for the free-hand drawings, photographs or charts that are used for documentation. Before the arrival of computers, graphics had to be drawn or created professionally to be suitable for publication. Now special computer programs have

replaced humans in the production of graphics for use in publishable medical articles.

What the author(s) believe the results of the study mean is not presented to readers in this section, but in the Discussion section.

## Discussion

This section, written in the present tense, describes to readers what the author(s) believe the findings described in the Results section actually mean. The purpose of the Discussion section is to tell readers the answers to the questions originally posed by the study, to discuss the significance of the results obtained by doing the study, and to relate these findings to previously published relevant studies, if any. From a structural standpoint, a good Discussion section begins by answering the question(s) that originally stimulated the study. The author(s) next present the evidence produced by the study that supports both answers to the original question(s) and the declaration by the author(s) of their significance. This section ends with a discussion of the significance of the evidence produced by the study that supports answers to both the original question(s) asked and the declaration by the author(s) of their significance. Physician writers must concentrate on showing the relationship(s) among observed facts and only discuss the significance of these facts in the Discussion section. The length of the Discussion section may vary depending upon the complexity of the topic and the observed results, the amount of evidence presented to readers, and the number of important points that need to be discussed. There is no set rule that governs the length of the Discussion section. It should be of sufficient length to give the physician author(s) an opportunity to convince readers and reviewers that the arguments supporting the conclusions and the significance of the results obtained in the study are clear, logical and reasonable. As is also true of the Results section, the Discussion section tests the physician writer's ability to discriminate among a mass of collected information. Readers must simply be presented with the facts and figures needed to support and justify the conclusions of the study as reported by the author(s).

The essential points of a good Discussion section can be summarized as follows.

1  Present the principles, relationships and generalizations contained in the Results section. Discuss, but do not recapitulate, the Results section.

2 Point out to readers any exceptions or lack of correlation in the findings of the study, and define any unsettled points in the text.
3 Show how the results of the study and their interpretation(s) agree or contrast with previously published work.
4 Discuss the theoretical implications of the study results as well as any practical applications, such as the possible clinical relevance of the findings.
5 State the conclusions of the study and the supporting data as clearly as possible.
6 Summarize the evidence for each conclusion drawn from the study results.
7 Discuss the significance of the presented conclusions.
8 Point out the potential areas for additional study and the possible implications for the clinical practice of medicine, or for medicine's related disciplines.

It needs to be pointed out that most inexperienced physician writers seem to experience greatest difficulty with the Discussion section. This is the section in which physician writers must present their arguments concerning the validity and meaning of the data obtained in the study, and the correctness of the derived conclusions. Physician writers must remember that argument is the art of persuasion, and it is the reader whom the physician writer should be persuading with regard to the validity and correctness of the physician writer's position. Physician writers are more likely to be successful in persuading readers to adopt their stated positions if they present their evidence in logically developed arguments expressed in clear and simple language. A frequent error made by inexperienced physician writers is to use the Discussion section to extrapolate the meaning of their data far beyond what is warranted by the evidence presented to readers in the text. Unfortunately, this extrapolation is often expressed in sentences of sweeping speculation that are certain to incur both the wrath of the medical journal editor and a liberal dose of their red pencil.

There is one cardinal rule that physician writers must follow when using this or any other established writing format. When composing text under one of these specific manuscript sections, the physician writer must stick to the subject matter defined by the format heading. For example, a description of results obtained in the study must be confined to the Results section and not be scattered among the other sections. This rule is absolute because readers use the journal's format to find the kind of information in which they might have a particular interest. Physician writers must therefore follow this journal format exactly so that their written articles can be separated by readers into distinct and different sections, each with its own purpose and content. Appropriate use of this writing format allows the information contained in the written article to be more understandable, useful and accessible to medical journal readers. Physician writers must also understand and accept graciously the fact that medical readers generally remember the content material of a good and worthwhile article, but rarely remember the name(s) of the physician writer(s).

Although encountered less frequently now in medical journals, the format of some basic science journals may still require a Conclusion section in the submitted paper. If required by a particular journal, the Conclusion section summarizes the questions that generated the study, the evidence produced by doing the study, and the answers framed by the data produced by the research undertaken, and may elaborate on any possible clinical relevance or technical application of the reported basic science results. However, in the usual type of clinical article, this type of final summation belongs in the Discussion section, thus making the need for a Conclusion section superfluous.

## Bibliography

There are two useful ways to keep track of references when writing an article for possible publication.

1  Make and retain a photocopy of the entire text of each article that the physician writer might plan to use as a reference to be cited in the final form of the article.
2  List all pertinent information about selected and possible reference sources on index cards and save them in a binder for possible future use in the completed article.

Physician authors should always follow the reference style and form preferred by selected journals as listed in the journal's Instructions for Authors. List only significant published references in the order preferred by the selected journal. Identify as "in press" articles cited in the Bibliography section that have been accepted for publication by a reputable journal, but have not yet been published. In general, references to unpublished data, personal communications, abstracts, theses and other secondary sources are not considered appropriate for inclusion in a bibliography of an article that is being prepared for submission to a peer-reviewed medical or scientific journal. Authors must check all parts of every reference cited against the original article to ensure accuracy of the citation before submitting the completed manuscript for editorial review and possible publication. References cited in a book or in another published medical article may be used by physician writers to provide adequate background information to readers, and must be selected carefully for their support and relevance to the material being presented to readers. References give life and vitality to points made in the written text, and must be carefully selected by physician writers. Medical journal editors regard an accurate listing of references in the submitted manuscript as an extremely important part of the completed article. Depending upon the preference of the selected medical journal, citation numbers can be placed directly following the name of the cited author(s), or added at the end of the sentence. The authors of medical articles must also make certain that the references chosen for use in the article are formatted in the form preferred by the selected journal. If the author(s) submit an article for editorial review that follows the format of another medical journal, the medical editor and manuscript reviewers might assume that the submitted article they are reviewing was previously rejected by another journal. Responsibility for the accuracy of references belongs to and remains with the submitting author(s). It is not the business of a journal editor or reviewer to check the accuracy of submitted references in an article that is undergoing editorial review.

## Revising a First Draft

Any physician writer who is satisfied with the first draft of their manuscript is either extraordinarily talented, or needs to immediately raise their writing standards. Revising and rewriting what has been written is an exercise that physician authors should carry out in a continuous fashion during the writing process in order to make certain that what has been written has been stated with accuracy, clarity, brevity and as much grace as possible. Later drafts of material written by physicians generally read better than earlier drafts, because good physician writers think hard about what they have written and the prose they have created with a view to making it better, and this includes correcting all misspellings. This thinking process allows ideas to develop gradually, resulting in better organization and structure of the material, clearer sentence formation, or more appropriate word choices as the revision work progresses. The best way to shorten an article is to delete all irrelevancies and needless repetitions in the written material. Once the physician writer has developed the ability to write their material for the reader, and has developed sufficient writing skills to be able to direct their material to a reader, they will then be well on the way to becoming a better physician writer. Although writing in medicine basically deals with medical and health-related factual information, the physician writer should try to accomplish this result with as much grace and style as possible in the writing.

## Summary: Medical Writing for Publication

At all times follow the instructions published in the Information for Authors section of the selected journal. Learn and use the writing technique known as technical writing. Use the IMRAD format when organizing and writing medical articles. This organizational format allows medical articles to be organized in logically derived sequences that are disciplined and easily recognized by readers and medical journal reviewers. These specific sections can be summarized as follows.

- The Introduction section tells readers what problem is under study, or what question the physician writer wishes to answer. It is written in the present tense because it is describing actions that are going on at present.
- The Materials and Methods section tells readers how the described problem was solved, or how the question posed in the Introduction was answered. This section is written in the past tense because the information given was compiled in the past.
- The Results section tells readers what was discovered as a result of doing the study, and is written in the past tense because it describes findings determined in the past.
- In the Discussion section the authors tell readers what they believe their findings mean. This section is always written in the present tense.

The package that the author(s) send to the editor of the selected journal must include the appropriate number of duplicate manuscript copies and accompanying graphics, along with a letter of transmittal. Details about information that must be contained in the transmittal letter can be found in the Instructions for Authors section in the selected journal. The letter of transmittal is usually written by the principal author, but in some instances all of the co-authors may be required to sign it. The journal will require one author to be specifically identified as the corresponding author for purposes of correspondence. Most medical journals require a letter of transmittal to include a statement on authorship responsibility, which means that all listed co-authors contributed to some extent to the planning, design and data collection for the study and the writing of the submitted manuscript. Authors must also disclose the source of any funds they have received to assist in the study and in the writing of the manuscript. In addition, the transmittal letter must contain an agreement from the author(s) to transfer, assign or convey to the journal all copyright ownership pertaining to the submitted article in the event that the journal agrees to publish the submitted manuscript. When submitting a manuscript to a medical journal, the author(s) must also make a full disclosure to the journal editor of any submissions and prior reports that could be regarded as prior or duplicate publications of the same or similar work.

Once the submitted article has arrived in the journal editor's office, the peer review process by the journal editor and perhaps several associate editors begins. Most medical journals will send the corresponding author notification of the manuscript's arrival in the journal office. Physician writers must understand that peer review of submitted manuscripts is a necessary part of good medical writing. Good peer review prevents the publication of bad work, improves scholarship, and improves both the language used by the physician writer(s) and the presentation of the data. Following completion of the peer review process, the author(s) are notified, by mail or email, of the journal's decision, which could be acceptance for publication, editorial suggestions for improvement of the text, or rejection of the manuscript for publication. Rejected manuscripts are rarely returned to the author(s), so physician writers must be certain to retain a copy of the submitted manuscript in their possession.

## Responding to a Rejection Letter from a Journal Editor

Physician writers must understand and accept the fact that medical journal editors are not advocates for writers, but rather they are advocates for readers. Put another way, medical journal editors are friends to readers but are not necessarily friends to physician writers who have submitted articles to their journal. Rejection letters from most medical journals will inform the author(s) of the journal's reasons for rejecting the manuscript for publication. If the reasons cite serious defects, such as questioning the validity of the science, or point out that the author's conclusions are not substantiated by the evidence presented, or inform the author(s) that similar material has been published previously, then the submitting author(s) may be out of luck. However, if the author(s) believe that the editor or manuscript reviewer misinterpreted or misunderstood the topic, the data presented or the conclusions drawn, they have every right to ask the journal editor to review the submitted manuscript again. A request for a second review should be made in a letter to the journal editor with accompanying documentation supporting the request for a second editorial review. One reason for manuscript rejection could be that the selected journal was not an appropriate choice of medical journal for the topic under consideration.

If the rejection letter is final and offers no hope of editorial softening to the physician writer, the author(s) should revise the article in accordance with the editorial criticisms offered in the letter of rejection. After these revisions have been completed, the manuscript can be sent to another journal in the physician writer's field of competence, probably a slightly less prestigious journal than the one selected initially. It is quite appropriate to keep sending the manuscript to other journals until the physician author either succeeds in getting the manuscript published, or runs out of appropriate journals in their field of competence. However, it is not acceptable to send the manuscript to more than one journal at a time. Physician writers should not get unduly upset by the arrival of a rejection letter from a medical journal. There are probably few published physician writers who have not received at least one rejection letter from some medical journal during their writing careers. Instead of becoming overly discouraged, physician writers should work hard to improve both their writing and organizational skills and to strengthen the breadth and significance of the data being reported, and successful publication should follow eventually.

Chapter 6

# Conferences and Talks: Presentation and Publication

For many physicians, delivering oral presentations to peers rates as an unwelcome task. Yet oral presentations can be among the most effective ways to present medical information to peers and to the public.[10] Writing and speaking are powerful and persuasive forms of medical communication, and physicians should be encouraged to broaden and improve their skills in the techniques of both forms of communication. However, the two types of human communication differ widely in their manner of presentation. It is also important for physicians to understand that these two forms of communication with other physicians and patients have different characteristics, because the written word is much more formal than is the spoken word. There is a need for physicians to not only be aware of the structural and stylistic differences between written and spoken language, but also to understand and appreciate how each form of medical communication can be used most effectively. Presenting a medical conference or delivering a medical talk before a professional audience provides the medical speaker with a unique opportunity to transfer useful information from his or her mind directly to the minds of a listening audience. In stark contrast to medical writing, presenting medical conferences and giving talks to a listening medical audience allows the physician speaker greater freedom of personal expression with regard to how the material is organized and presented. This is because the major elements of this form of medical communication are less structured than the elements required for publishable medical writing. This form of medical communication is based on conversation, the most familiar form of human communication, and is a form of communication that is used by physicians every day.[11]

Physicians who wish to be more effective in commanding the attention of medical audiences in order to move them toward the positions advocated by their spoken messages can accomplish this by learning and using the techniques developed for medical speaking. In contrast to medical writing, medical speaking allows a greater freedom of personal expression in how the material is presented because content, organization and delivery – the major elements of this form of medical communication – are less restrictive than the elements required for successful medical writing. The ability to speak effectively and deliver a message that is both useful to and remembered by a listening audience rests on good organization and preparation of the talk, knowing something of the interests of the audience and their familiarity with the subject matter, and presenting the spoken material to the listening audience in an interesting way. When preparing material for oral presentation to a listening audience, physician speakers must be alert to possible differing levels of audience familiarity with the subject matter of the presentation, so that efforts can be made to keep the attention of the entire audience throughout the oral presentation.

When readers find a written passage unclear, they can review the writing again at their own pace until they understand what has been written. If their attention lapses they can return to the item at any time to refresh their memories about the unclear part of the written material. However, when part of a medical talk is unclear or confuses some of the listening audience, they may well remain bewildered and, as a consequence, stop listening and gain nothing from the oral presentation.

In oral medical presentations more than in any other form of medical communication, special attention is required from the speaker to keep the presented material clear and interesting so that all members of the audience can understand and follow the development of the points and ideas that are being presented. The use of first- rather than third-person pronouns and the active rather than the passive voice will contribute to a smoother, more informal speaking style that will be appreciated by a listening audience. The effect of the talk, and any benefit derived from it by the listening audience, will depend greatly on the physician speaker's personality, motivation, speaking voice and style of delivery, and on the value of the presented material to the listening audience.

Regardless of whether the physician speaker decides to use a prepared text or notes, or speak from projected graphic material, their speaking style and delivery should be factual and objective without being dry, boring and uninteresting to the listening audience. Physician speakers should never lose sight of the fact that they are speaking to an audience of their peers who have an interest in the material that the speaker is about to present to them. This is where the personal style of the physician speaker comes into play, with judicious and naturally appearing humor when the situation indicates, and the occasional gesture, while at the same time avoiding the appearance of being pretentious or lecturing the audience. Speak slowly, clearly and loudly enough for everyone in the audience to be able to hear the spoken words without having to strain. Physician speakers who speak too quickly, or who use a low speaking voice, risk losing the attention of their audiences within a very short time. Physician speakers must work to perfect the technique of speaking effectively from prepared texts and, above all else, must resist the temptation to simply read the text to the listening audience. The most critical technique to master is to learn how to transfer vocally useful information to an audience both effectively and clearly. Regardless of the size of the audience, the location of the setting or the prominence of the meeting, success in the endeavor for the physician speaker rests upon having good material to present, good organization and preparation of the material to be presented, interesting graphics, and a pleasing style of delivery of the material during the presentation. A pleasing delivery style is enhanced by good vocal tone and appropriate use of voice modulation where appropriate.

The form of the delivered talk is essential to clarity for the audience. Regardless of whether the speaker's decision is to use a prepared text, notes, or speak from projected graphic material, the information given in the talk will be received best by the listening audience if the material is presented in a logically organized format consisting of three stages as follows.

1  Present the reasons for giving the talk.
2  Present the data supporting the physician speaker's position.
3  Explain carefully to the audience what the speaker believes the presented information means.

A good stage presence and appearance by the physician speaker can help to make the message more convincing to a listening audience. Although few physicians are naturally gifted speakers, most can master the oral techniques that will enable them to speak with authority and confidence. As physicians gain experience with this form of medical communication, most will develop an individual speaking style appropriate to their own personality. A distinction worth noting has been made between an experienced speaker and a good speaker. It is said that an experienced speaker goes on making the same mistakes, but with increasing confidence. However, a good speaker is one who asks friends and colleagues to tell him or her what was wrong with the presentation so that mistakes can be corrected.

Physician speakers should always try to compose an opening message that gets the immediate attention of the audience. Consider the effectiveness of the opening two sentences that Daniel Webster used when he rose in the US Senate, on March 7, 1850, to join the debate on the Clay Compromise. He began, "I speak today for the preservation of the Union. Hear me for my cause." Simplicity, repetition and alliteration in the text and vocal cadence and tone modulation in the delivery are more effective in oral presentations than are long sentences and big words. Regardless of how knowledgeable physician speakers may be about their subject matter, those speakers who fail to impose structure on their text will ramble when delivering it, and will dilute the message intended for the listening audience and risk losing the attention of that audience.

Physicians who have to prepare a text for oral presentation before a medical audience of any size would do well to reflect on the words contained in a memorandum sent to young reporters by Edward R Murrow, a renowned World War Two journalist: "First, you tell them what you are going to tell them. Then you tell them. Then you tell them what you told them." What this quote is telling physician speakers is that the most critical speaking technique to master is learning how to transfer useful medical information to a listening audience effectively, simply and clearly.

Unless the physician speaker has a deep and thorough grasp of their subject matter, the best way for most speakers to make an effective oral presentation is to speak from a prepared text. Print the text in large upper-case letters with double or triple spacing which gives the physician speaker the opportunity to add handwritten notes on personal speaking instructions. Notations can be added to the text pages about the use of illustrative materials. However, physicians must work to perfect the technique of speaking effectively to a listening audience from prepared texts and, above all else, must resist the temptation to simply read the text to a listening professional audience. The most critical technique to master is how to vocally transfer useful information to a listening professional audience effectively and clearly, with style and grace.

## Points to Remember about Delivering a Talk

1 With a typed or printed and appropriately marked text in front of the speaker, the circumstances governing the talk should be under the physician speaker's control.
2 Speak in a voice that is loud enough to be easily heard by the entire audience, speak clearly and pronounce words distinctly, and use a speaking cadence that is geared to the time period allotted for the presentation.
3 Time the talk carefully during practice sessions so that you can make effective use of the allotted time period. Exceeding the allotted time period is bad speaking manners and may result in the microphone being turned off. Exceeding your time limit also may encroach on the time allotted to the next speaker, thus possibly causing them to lose time from their presentation.
4 Use your nervous energy constructively. Project your voice and your message to the audience in the back row of the auditorium.
5 Look at the audience as much as possible when presenting the talk (80% of the time is believed reasonable). Making strong eye contact with the audience suggests to them that the speaker has confidence and control.
6 Make any gestures, such as using a pointer, in full view of the audience. If you have to move away from the microphone, make sure that you are wearing a lapel microphone, and under no circumstances just wander around the podium in a purposeless fashion.
7 For a positive and forceful conclusion to the talk, memorize the last few sentences of the text. Deliver them with the room lights on and while looking at the audience. Pause for a few seconds after finishing the talk and continue to look at the audience. Thank the audience for their attention, field any questions that may come from them, gather your notes together and sit down.

Medical speakers should always conclude their talks by reviewing with the audience the points that were made in the talk, and by explaining their meaning and relevance to the practice of medicine, so as to leave the audience with a sense of closure and direction. Speakers can signal the approach of the end of the talk by using phrases such as "in summary" or "in conclusion." Such phrases tend to sharpen the attention of listeners to focus on what the physician speaker is about to say. The most effective oral presentations end with a clear and concise summary of the conclusions derived from the presented material. Summation points should be delivered to the audience with the room lights on and with the physician speaker again in eye contact with the audience. The best advice for physician speakers is to come to the lectern fully prepared and with a well-organized and well-rehearsed talk. A clear and measured speaking style and delivery, and the showing of useful illustrations, will help to add to the professionalism of the presentation, but will in no way substitute for preparation, organization, and practice in giving talks to professional audiences.

## Converting a Talk into a Possible Publication

Organizing and writing the text for a medical talk follows a quite different format from that used for organizing and writing text for possible publication in a medical journal. Texts written for possible publication are rather rigidly structured and follow a generally accepted and a more formal publication format. Unlike text for published medical articles, orally delivered texts are written for the ears of listeners and must be delivered to listening audiences in such a way that the important points made in the orally delivered material can be heard, understood clearly and remembered by a listening audience. Texts written for oral delivery are rarely interchangeable with texts written for possible publication in medical journals. There are specific and non-interchangeable differences between spoken and written material, and neither can be substituted for the other without substantial rewriting. Physicians who wish to attempt to change an orally presented text into a text that might be suitable for possible publication in a medical journal would be well advised to reread Chapters 3, 4 and 5 before beginning the effort.

Talks given by physicians rarely contain enough new and significant information to attract the attention of medical journal editors. Occasionally, however, a physician may present enough new and significant material, which if rewritten in the approved writing format could attract the attention of a medical journal editor. Such physicians must understand at the outset that this type of information transformation is not easy and will require substantial reworking and rewriting of the text material. Before beginning this arduous exercise, the physician must be certain that he or she fully understands the differences in presentation and format between spoken material and written material. Organizing and writing the text for a medical talk follows quite a different format from that used for organizing and writing an article for possible publication. Texts for possible publication are rather rigidly structured and follow a generally accepted publishing format. Unlike text for published medical articles, orally delivered texts are written for the ears of the audience and must be delivered to the listening audience in such a way that the important points presented in the orally delivered text can be heard, understood clearly and remembered by the audience. Texts written for oral presentation are therefore rarely interchangeable with texts written for publication.

The challenge facing medical speakers who wish to convert their material that has been written for a talk into a possible publication is to repackage the material from the talk into a form that is more suitable for possible publication in a medical journal. The following five steps are involved in this process.

1  Read and follow the advice given in Chapter 5.
2  Use the writing form known as technical writing (*see* Chapter 3).
3  Redirect the text from its auditory focus (material that is delivered vocally) to a visual focus (material that is read).
4  Change the structure of the material in the talk from a speaking format of Introduction, Body of Material and Conclusions to the writing format of Introduction, Materials and Methods, Results and Discussion.
5  Add the following material.
   • Add a statement of purpose at the end of the Introduction, to provide readers with a brief, clear expression of the purpose of performing and reporting the study in question.
   • Add a full explanation of the study design in the Materials and Methods section.
   • Add a full explanation of the study findings in the Results section.
   • Use only the most relevant tables, graphs and illustrations. A Medical Media service at a medical school or at a large general hospital will be equipped to convert computer-assisted illustrations into photographs suitable for publication in a medical journal.
   • Add a bibliography.

- Always follow the advice and requirements listed in the selected journal's Instructions for Authors.
- Ask a well-published medical colleague to review the completed text for appropriate comments before sending the manuscript to a journal for editorial review.

Text for publication in a medical journal must be written for the benefit of readers, not for a listening audience, which means that the physician writer must deliver a clear and logical presentation of the evidence derived from the study, a clear presentation of the arguments in support of the presented evidence, and a clear presentation of the conclusions resulting from the evidence derived from the study. The text should be written in a simple and spare style and be free from medical jargon, unfamiliar terms, eponyms and abbreviations. Medical writing for publication must be constructed in language that is grammatically correct, simple in its construction, clear in its meaning to readers, and pleasing to read. Good physician writing is a combination of good material or data, good vocabulary, good sentence structure and good organization of the presented data or material.

Four guiding principles can help physicians to plan, organize and write a text derived from a talk for possible publication in a medical journal.

1  Develop a different sense of audience, which now means to write for a reader rather than for a listening audience. Stop the writing every few pages and assume the role of a reader to make certain that what has been written will be clearly understandable to readers. Ask colleagues to read what has been written and comment on its readability.
2  Recognize that medical writing is a form of technical writing. The physician writer must be clear about the differences between technical writing and literary writing, because the two writing forms differ greatly in orientation and purpose in the writing effort.
3  Never forget that the real danger of careless and imprecise medical writing is the transfer of careless and imprecise information about a piece of potentially important and useful material to medical readers, which may have an unfortunate impact on the health of people. The physician writer must work to develop writing discrimination, which is the need to develop an appropriate sense of content of the projected material, covering what to include as well as what to exclude. Writing discrimination tends to develop with writing experience, but its development can be helped along by

thinking about the writing as the writing progresses. Most inexperienced physician writers show their lack of writing discrimination by filling their manuscripts with every piece of information they can dredge up from their preparatory study or work-up. In addition, physician writers must always studiously avoid the temptation to fall in love with their own words.

4   Use the writing form known as technical writing (*see* Chapter 3) when constructing text for possible publication. The material to be used in a possible journal article should be written in plain, clear language and must be written with the constant needs of readers, not listeners, foremost in the physician writer's mind. The need for absolute clarity in medical writing stems from a principal axiom of good medical writing: never assume that a potential medical reader knows everything about the subject matter of the written materials.

Chapter 7

# Grant Writing

Grant money for worthy research projects is available from foundations of various kinds, the National Institutes of Health (NIH), and occasionally from corporations of various kinds.[12] The first requirement facing a grant applicant is to make certain that the content material and emphasis of the proposed research application, as defined in the grant application, match the purposes, goals and special interests of the funding source from whom money for the proposed research project is being requested. For example, there are approximately 24,000 private foundations that provide money to support research projects. However, foundations vary in size and have differing purposes, goals and special interests that determine for whom and for what purposes they will award grant funds for reviewed research projects. Grant applicants who solicit foundations for research support must therefore first be certain that their grant request is tailored to reflect the special interests of the particular selected foundation.

One of the main functions of the NIH is to award funds to outside investigators in support of biomedical research. The majority of NIH grant awards are in the form of investigator-initiated research project grant applications (coded ROI by NIH), regardless of whether the grant application is for support of a proposed basic science or clinical research study. Other types of grant awards exist at NIH, and information about obtaining NIH grants can be obtained from the Division of Research Grants at NIH. Applying for NIH grant funding is a difficult, demanding and time-consuming process because the NIH Grant Application Form imposes very strict guidelines on the structure and format of the grant application material.[13] In addition to good science, applicants for NIH grant funding must present a well-organized and well-written grant proposal. The form for the application itself is strictly constrained with regard to page length, so close attention to detail is required from the grant application writer. If the application is for a clinical study, statistical support is essential and the experimental plan must document methods for patient accrual and numbers of patients required to meet specific statistical objectives. It is also important for grant application writers to demonstrate sound procedures for data collection, management of the data, and an accurate analysis of the collected data in the grant application. Brevity, clarity and organization in the writing of the application are essential components of a successful NIH grant application.

Grant application writing requires a particularly lucid, precise and organized writing style because the purpose of applying for a grant is to ask for money to support a proposed research project. Two issues are paramount in writing grant proposals, namely having something worthwhile to say to a grant funding source along with supporting data, and saying it clearly and succinctly.[14] Money to support medical research projects can come from a variety of sources, including departmental or institutional funds, occasionally from corporations, foundations of many types, and government sources such as the NIH. However, all funding sources, regardless of type, have specific and often different purposes, goals and special interests which are fundamental to their reasons for supporting appropriate medical research projects. These individual differences in goals, purposes and grant request requirements make it mandatory for physician researchers who are planning to seek research funding support to make it their business to learn about the specific requirements of all appropriate funding sources before beginning the process of grant application writing. A summary of these specific requirements can be requested from potential funding sources. Physicians who are requesting grant funds for research projects need to understand that grant money is not in endless supply in this country. In order to be successful in obtaining grant funding, the writing of the grant application becomes paramount.

The first requirement facing a grant applicant is to make certain that the content, purpose, goals and emphasis of the planned research project, as defined in the grant application, match the purposes, goals and special interests of the funding source from whom the grant money is being requested. Before awarding research funds, most funding sources will require answers to three basic questions:

1 information about the principal investigator (the research background of the principal investigator, such as their educational and research background, research achievements to date, etc.)

2  what the investigator wants to do with the money (outline of proposed research project)
3  how much money is needed to accomplish the goals of the research project.

Answers to these and other questions asked by the funding source make up the content material relating to the proposed research project that is detailed in the body of the grant application. How well and how persuasively this content material is presented in the grant application will reflect the writing and organizational skills of the grant application writer. The chances of success in obtaining grant funding support are improved by including within the details of the grant application a previously performed pilot study, or other completed original research studies.

Because the demand for research funding far exceeds the amount of money currently available, grant applicants can increase their chances of success by submitting interesting, well-organized and well-written grant proposals. Grant application writing calls for straightforward and concise language that incorporates appropriate technical terms. The submitted grant application must focus on a solid objective and must be supported by a clear and concise plan for its successful accomplishment. Trying to pursue multiple hypotheses or solve all possible problems in a single grant application weakens the grant application and increases the likelihood of rejection of the proposal. Diffuseness in organizing and writing grant applications and a lack of focus in the research plan are other major reasons why many grant applications are not approved for funding by the funding source. Successful grant applications clearly and persuasively describe what questions, issues or hypotheses are to be addressed, what the principal investigator and other researchers have accomplished in previous research efforts leading up to the current research project, how the research will be carried out, and for how long financial support will be required to bring the research project to a definitive conclusion in a reasonable time frame. Grant money allocated by educational, governmental or philanthropic organizations must only be used for these purposes unless the granting agency gives the researchers specific permission for a reallocation of the grant funds.

The writing of a grant application must follow the instructions and guidelines for the format and content of the grant proposal as stated by the funding source. The style and format of good grant applications combine good writing skills with a clear writing style, and a feasible and clearly presented research plan. The content material of successful grant applications begins with a good research idea, and approaches the answers to the proposed questions with good medical science. The underlying good idea and good medical science contained in the grant application must come from each investigator's creativity and research skills. Hypothesis-generated research that is directed toward an important clinical or scientific mechanism of action is often most successful in obtaining funding. Demonstrating the capability for successfully accomplishing the proposed research study is the responsibility of the grant applicant, and it must be shown in the strength and persuasiveness of the grant application. The grant application must contain enough preliminary data to satisfy even the most skeptical of grant reviewers that the grant applicant has the knowledge, skills and ability to carry out a full-scale research project to a successful conclusion. Previously published research results, preliminary data obtained from previous research or a recently completed pilot study, and identification of appropriate and knowledgeable collaborators are also helpful elements of a successful grant application. The grant application must deliver a strong and clear message to grant reviewers that the proposed research project as described in the application can be done and is worth doing. A complete and well-written grant application provides grant reviewers with a clear focus on the hypothesis and research plan, and an appreciation of the logical and scientific approach needed to accomplish the goals of the proposed research as outlined in the grant application.

In grant terms, the lead investigator is called the principal investigator and, in addition to being the lead investigator, he or she also carries the responsibility for making certain that the grant application is written with great care and follows the writing instructions issued by the grant funding source. A poorly written description of the proposed research project, an error in adding up the budget, or an unclear graph of the preliminary results could easily lead to rejection of the grant application. The principal investigator of a basic science or clinical medical research grant application is also responsible for the writing of the grant application, as well as for proposing, designing and reporting the research results. The principal investigator may delegate portions of the preparation work for the grant application to others involved with the study, but this delegation of authority does not relieve the principal investigator of responsibility for the conduct of these other individuals. Inexperienced grant application writers should seek advice and help about the content matter and budget of the grant application from other more experienced colleagues. The principal investigator and the grant proposal writer, if they are different individuals, must both be involved with the budget process so that possible questions asked by the funding source about how the budget relates to the proposed research can be answered fully and appropriately.

The grant applicant must be certain that the proposed grant budget is completely justified and is commensurate with the scope and relevance of the projected research study. Grant reviewers are too sophisticated and knowledgeable not to recognize and reject artificially inflated budgets. Conversely, a budget that seems too modest for the proposed research project may suggest to grant reviewers that the grant applicant has poor judgment. The grant applicant must be certain that appropriate indirect costs are included in the submitted grant budget figures. Indirect costs are the additional sums added to the grant budget to support administrative and maintenance costs incurred by the grant applicant's institution. These costs add a fixed percentage of the total requested budget for the research project to the total budget request. The size of the percentage to be added for indirect costs is determined by the grant applicant's institution.

Grant applicants should plan sufficient time to be able to write multiple drafts and to receive preliminary reviews of the proposed grant application and its writing from interested colleagues with positive grant request histories. This must all be done prior to the deadline for submitting the grant application to the funding source. In general, sources for data can be cited in the body of the grant application, but footnotes and unsupported assumptions must be avoided. The original proposal should be sent to the funding source, but only include duplicate copies if the funding source requests them. Extravagant proposal packaging should be avoided. An unusual proposal format or packaging risks focusing more attention on the form of the proposal than on its substance, and may suggest to the funding source that the applicant has a tendency to waste money.

If the submitted grant proposal for funding is rejected, the rejection notice often comes with a request for more data, a requested reply from the grant applicant to specific objections made by the grant reviewer to the purpose of the proposal, or suggestions for a revised approach to the study from the grant reviewer, which in essence is an invitation to try again. A grant applicant whose grant request is rejected initially by the funding source should respond to the criticisms or suggestions offered by the grant reviewer and, after making the suggested changes, resubmit the improved grant application.

Although this has not been documented, the chances of receiving funding for a proposed research project appear to increase each time a grant application is improved and resubmitted for funding consideration, because it seems that most granting agencies tend to regard tenacity in grant application writers as a virtue.

Chapter 8

# Improved Physician Communication Skills

In addition to being able to give effective talks at medical meetings and being talented enough to be able to write medical articles that are acceptable for publication by medical journals, physicians also need appropriate communication skills to allow them to discuss worrisome medical problems with patients in a clear and forthright manner. "My doctor doesn't talk to me" and "My doctor doesn't tell me anything about my condition" are complaints frequently voiced by patients about their own doctors. Other patients, for a variety of different reasons, appear to be reluctant to ask many questions of their physician about their medical problem. Insightful physicians pick up this patient reluctance and gently question the patient about his or her understanding of the discussed medical problem and its proposed treatment.

Good relationships between doctors and patients have long been recognized as critical alliances by the medical profession, but now seem to be honored more frequently in the breach than in the doing by some physicians. A belief persists among some patients that inter-personal problems arising between physicians and patients are aggra-vated by a sense that some physicians seem to overemphasize curing at the expense of caring. Too often physicians regard the art of medicine, bedside manner and "people skills" with suspicion because the scientific basis for these important interpersonal interactions seems to lack the objectivity of René Laënnec, the eighteenth-century French physician credited with inventing the stethoscope. He reput-edly advised his physician nephew that, even though doctors might think it silly, doctors hold their credit solely from the public and it would be foolish for young doctors not to respect this role of the public. Although empathy toward patients is recognizable in physicians who possess this quality, empirical investigation of physician empathy is scarce because of conceptual ambiguity and the lack of a psychometrically sound tool for measuring physician empathy.[15]

Some hospitals and medical centers are now beginning to ask their patients to rate their physician's communication skills and availability, as well as the technical aspects of the care that they received as patients. This becomes a new and compelling reason for physicians to take stock of their patient communication and interpersonal skills. In truth, medical practice needs to become more socially conscious and responsive to the needs of its patients. This calls for a shift from the paternalistic "doctor knows best" model of medical care to a more egalitarian model characterized by the consent process and shared decision making. Knowing what is best for patients remains an accepted reason for physicians to act on their behalf, provided that patients are fully informed of the reasons for the physician's actions and are offered the opportunity to become part of the decision-making process and to have their medical questions answered satisfactorily by their physician.

Some medical institutions now even include provisions for added physician reimbursements, or bonuses, tied to performance targets set by the medical institution. Incentive bonus plans offered to participating physicians by these organizations are usually tied to the score obtained by rating physicians on patient satisfaction, perceived quality of offered medical care, and cost-effectiveness. Physicians who constantly receive low scores on these hospital-imposed criteria may not only be denied bonus payments, but could also lose patients through these arbitrary criteria. This certainly should be motivation enough for physicians to make sure that they learn more about good people skills and how to make better use of those skills.

The medical profession has always regarded communication and interpersonal skills as necessary attributes for physicians, and the ability to interact well with sick patients has been a widely held goal of medical education for years. Indeed, human communication is believed by many physician educators to be an essential component of the physician's role. However, many patients now do not believe that physicians do a good job either in communicating information to them about their health problems, or in expressing concern about their welfare as patients. The available evidence suggests that poor physician communication and poor interpersonal skills are neither a new phenomenon nor a specific by-product of medical practice, but rather they represent personal deficiencies that have persisted in many physicians since their medical school days. Medical students and residents need help with communication skills, particularly in obtaining a good medical history from a patient, conveying clear and accurate information about diagnosis and treatment to patients and their families, reassuring sick patients, achieving patient compliance with advised treatment plans, and monitoring how patients and their families adapt to illness and to its treatment. Many physicians have been found to lack the ability to adequately explain an illness to a patient, to determine a patient's level of understanding and emotional response to an illness, and to acquire an adequate social history from their patients.

It is probably unrealistic to expect that communication and interpersonal skills in medicine, if not acquired by students from their families or from past personal experiences, can be learned with sufficient intensity during a relatively short period of medical school education. It is even more difficult to learn these skills during the clinical years because, in most medical settings, the emphasis tends to be on the technical aspects of medical care rather than on the effect of the medical problem on the patient. Overwhelming responsibility for patients and the necessity for acquiring technical skills during the period of graduate medical education may, to some extent, act as a deterrent to the acquisition of effective communication and interpersonal skills for many young physicians during this period of their career development. To the extent that the practice of medicine has become more scientific and more dependent upon technology, the physician–patient relationship has been weakened. As the physician–patient relationship declines, so does physician availability and physician familiarity with the total patient. A frequently voiced complaint about the way in which medicine is now practiced is that touch has been replaced by technology. As physician author and historian, Kenneth Ludmerer, observes in *Time to Heal*, his classic book on American medical education in the twentieth century:

> the power of medical education is limited, particularly regarding its ability to produce doctors who are caring, socially responsible, and capable of behaving as patient advocates in all practice environments.[16]

In the light of these and other troublesome changes occurring in the medical practice environment, it seems both necessary and evident that physicians need to develop an improved professional image for themselves, and a more cordial relationship with their patients.

Professional pride in practice patterns and behaviors is an additional reason why physicians and patients need to communicate with each other more effectively. It has been shown in several studies that the way in which physicians communicate with patients has an effect on the accuracy of their diagnoses, the compliance of their patients with physician recommendations, and the responses and compliance of their patients with treatments and planned clinical investigations. The fact that patient satisfaction with their relationships with physicians correlates strongly with ratings for physician courtesy and information giving underscores the recommendation that the professional image of physicians in the eyes of patients would be greatly enhanced if physicians administered to themselves a large dose of common courtesy and common sense, along with the skills of information giving and listening to others.

A frequent criticism of physicians expressed by patients is that the rigorous scientific training required for their medical education depersonalizes some of them to the extent that effective medical technicians are produced who, upon entering the clinical practice of medicine, have fewer communication and interpersonal skills than they had upon entering medical school. Medical care in this instance can become system efficient but not patient oriented, and effective communication with patients suffers accordingly. It is also believed that as medical students become more and more focused on the medical problems associated with the human body, some of them become less focused on the person in the human body with the medical problem. In addition, personal relationships with patients can become attenuated and distorted by physicians depending too heavily on data reported by sources extraneous to both patient and physician. It has been shown that, on average, only about 10% of medical decisions for patients are made with the participation of a fully informed patient. Consequently, many of the interpersonal problems that arise from the physician–patient encounter are believed to be caused by a physician's perceived lack of balance between an emphasis on curing and an emphasis on caring which, when combined with the physician's inflated sense of importance and a dominant and directive attitude toward patients, can result in physician behavior that has been called ''the arrogance of expertise'' by some physician communication experts.

From the standpoint of physicians, a major and desirable goal of good physician–patient communication should be to improve the outcomes of patient care from the patient's perspective. The outcomes of diagnosis and medical treatment depend to a great extent on unimpaired communication between physicians and their patients. Failure to establish empathic relationships with patients can be a serious bar to good communication exchanges and to appropriate patient responses. Studies of patient complaints about doctors and malpractice claims show that malpractice actions appear mostly to be related to patient dissatisfaction with the physician's inability to establish rapport, provide access to them, administer care and treatment consistent with patient expectations, and to communicate with them effectively. The quality of rendered medical care depends to a great extent on the interactions between physicians and patients, and the suspicion exists that these kinds of interactions are all too frequently disappointing to both parties in the clinical dialogue. The more that patients actively participate in medical consultations about their care, the more likely they are to have better health care outcomes and quality of care. The strongest predictors of patient participation in their medical care are situation-specific, namely the clinical setting and the physician's communication style.[17]

As far as patients are concerned, the basic and possibly the most important type of communication with physicians, and the cornerstone upon which good medical care is built, is the interpersonal interaction between a physician and a patient. True compassion for the medical problems of patients is a by-product of sensitive and aware physician communication with patients. The absence of satisfying communication between physicians and patients thwarts physician medical skills and diminishes physician sensitivity to patient needs and concerns. The need for physicians to understand the problems associated with unsuccessful communication with patients and others is more important now than ever before, because the delivery of medical care is now more and more fragmented by specialized professionals and technicians, so that patients are increasingly forced to relate to a galaxy of different physicians and health care workers in their efforts to be relieved of their medical problems.

The clinical encounter is a complex interaction between a physician and a patient, both of whom have overlapping, but not entirely congruent, values and goals for the outcome of the encounter. How effective the outcome of the clinical encounter will be from the patient's perspective largely depends on the communication and interpersonal skills displayed by the treating physician. How a patient assesses the warmth displayed, the information given verbally and non-verbally about the medical problem under discussion, the laying on of hands, and other reassuring techniques employed by the physician during the clinical encounter generally reflects the professional attitude of the physician, as these attitudes relate to what has been called the art of medicine and bedside manner, both of which are components of good professional behavior. The key features of a good bedside manner shown by a physician have been described as a cheerful optimism with kindness, while engendering faith and hope in the patient and at the same time attempting to minimize the patient's pain and fear.

Although these are widely regarded as vital components of effective medical care, many practicing physicians continue to regard the art of medicine and bedside manner with suspicion and even disdain. Physician attitudes toward these vital components of good patient care mainly reflect their own beliefs that the scientific basis for these interpersonal interactions with patients lacks the precision and prestige of the bulk of scientific medicine. Consequently, each physician tends to have their own unique definition of what constitutes skill in relating to patients. Professional bias notwithstanding, physician communication with patients will not improve substantially until compassion, warmth, respect for and interest in patients as human beings begin to play a more prominent role in the physician–patient clinical interaction. Improvement in physician communication with patients and, consequently, improvement in the delivery of more effective and satisfying medical care to patients will require concerted actions by physicians, patients and others involved in the delivery of medical care in this country. Physicians and patients must value and respect each other for the needs and obligations that each brings to the clinical encounter.

Patients list kindness, understanding, interest in them as people, sympathy and encouragement as the most important attitudes that they wish their physician to possess. Patients evaluate a physician's attitude of caring by assessing the warmth, cordiality and courtesy extended to them by the physician. Patients evaluate a physician's competence and the quality of care provided to them by assessing the thoroughness that the physician displays during the clinical encounter, the use of preventive measures, and the physician's willingness and ability to share information with them about their medical problem. Patients frequently offer clues about their health concerns that can present opportunities for physicians to express sympathy and understanding about these patient health concerns. However, physicians too often tend to bypass these offered clues, thus missing opportunities to strengthen the physician–patient relationship. Patients are most satisfied with the communication interaction with their physician when the physician discovers and deals with the patient's concerns and expectations, when the physician's manner communicates warmth, interest and concern about the patient, and when the physician explains the medical situation to the patient in terms that can be understood by him or her. Consequently, patients want a physician whose attitude toward them creates trust and confidence, whose manner suggests thoroughness and concern, who allays their health-related tensions and fears, and who shows compassion by extending as much medical help to a fellow human being as it is possible to give.

It appears that patient cooperation with suggested treatment programs depends more on how the physician's communication skills are perceived by the patient than on anything else in the interaction. Patient satisfaction with a medical experience appears to be related more to the physician's skill as a patient communicator than to the perceived quality of the medical care received by or offered to the patient, the patient waiting time, or even the projected cost of the proposed medical treatment. An orientation statement by the physician to the patient at the beginning of the clinical encounter, such as "First I will examine you and then we will talk about the problem", can help to set the tone for a fruitful patient interview. Many patients complain that they are given little or inadequate information during a treatment phase of their illness, or while being treated at a hospital. A frequent patient complaint is that when physicians attempt to offer explanations to them about their illness or medical condition, these are difficult to understand because the physician frequently uses cryptic and obscure terms and medical jargon when giving medical explanations and medical instructions to patients. Medical jargon, also known as "medspeak", always confuses patients and never enlightens them.

It has become increasingly evident that how well or how poorly physicians communicate with their patients is of direct relevance to the accuracy of their diagnoses, and to the compliance, satisfaction with and response to treatment of their patients. The biggest barriers to good verbal communication between physicians and patients appear to include the use of medical jargon by physicians, an intimidating awe of physicians by some patients, and physicians who project to patients either verbally or non-verbally a perceived lack of time for them and hence a need to hurry through the clinical encounter with the patient. Although they are fluent in the jargon of their own medical specialty, physicians frequently cannot communicate easily with people outside the field of medicine, or occasionally even with physicians in other medical or surgical disciplines. Those physicians who treat patients with respect and who recognize the need to master the techniques of good communication skills are more likely to gather full and accurate information from their patients, to dispense clear and persuasive information to them and their families, and to elicit cooperation with the details of patient management plans from patients, their families and others involved in providing patient care.

All human communication behavior has as its purpose the elicitation of specific responses from a particular person or group of people. In order to become effective medical communicators, physicians must first understand the underlying purposes of communicating by either the spoken or written word. For physicians, effective communication with patients and others involves more skills than the mere giving of a message, not infrequently delivered in a stern authoritarian tone and in a time frame just short of being abrupt. Communication with others can be affected positively or negatively by the purpose and nature of the delivered message, the style or form in which it is delivered, the audience to whom the communication is addressed, the social, educational and cultural differences between the communicator and the recipient of the message – be it a single patient, a readership or a large professional audience – and the cheerfulness or lack of emotion with which the message is delivered.

The perception of the quality of the medical care delivered by physicians to patients depends largely on the assessment by patients of the quality of the human communication developed between them and their physicians. Patients are no longer impressed by physicians who spend their time looking at a computer screen during the patient interview, while the patient is attempting to describe their symptoms and reasons for consulting the doctor to the physician's back. Appropriate physician behavior when using an office computer during a patient visit should include the following.

1  The physician should describe to the patient what he or she is doing when typing or reviewing prior medical information from the computer screen.
2  The physician should avoid long periods of silence when at the computer, thus excluding the patient from the patient visit process.

3  The physician should maintain eye contact with the patient as often as possible when using a computer.
4  The physician must avoid sitting with their back to the patient when using a computer, mainly because it is rude behavior.

Physicians should recognize that the clinical information on their computer screen about patients can also be used as a teaching tool. Regardless of professional qualifications, physicians who are perceived by patients to be poor communicators are not regarded highly as caregivers by these patients. Effective communication with patients thus includes not only the outcomes desired by the message that is being communicated, but also the perception of satisfaction with the encounter experienced by both parties in the communication process.

Two additional dimensions of effective physician–patient communication relate to needs expressed by patients. The first need is for physicians to understand and appreciate patient concerns about the diagnosed illness or medical problem, including its cause, its severity, its prognosis, the results of provided tests and the availability of effective treatment. The other need is for the physician to give the patient the desired information about their illness and its possible treatment in clear and understandable language, and to be willing to answer any questions that the patient may have about the described illness. Unfortunately, some physicians now avoid this patient responsibility by substituting written material or videos for patient counseling, instead of face-to-face meetings with the patients. A critical component of an effective physician–patient interaction is the attentiveness displayed by the physician toward the information and non-verbal clues given by patients. Equally important to good physician–patient communication exchanges are the non-verbal clues expressed by physicians, who more often than not are unaware of expressing these clues, and are equally unaware of their effect on patients. Patients watch physicians' faces closely and are quite sensitive to the tone of voice employed by physicians when speaking with them. The physician's facial expression should reflect equanimity, and their speaking voice should be calm, friendly and clearly audible to patients. Physicians need to appreciate that empathy is the clinician's essential tool for understanding patients and their problems, and for selecting and reviewing appropriate treatment options with them.[18]

Physicians need to appreciate that information which is shared in an effective communication process initiates change in the behavior, thinking, lifestyle or attitude of the person receiving the information.

The communication process achieves its full potential when appropriate relationships exist or are developed among the communicators, the message being communicated, and the recipient of the communicated message. Communication is an interaction or relationship between human beings that involves the production of a spoken or written message by one individual and the receipt of that message by someone else. It is this ongoing process of sending and receiving messages that results in the creation of positive or negative communication relationships between humans. It is often the manner or style in which a spoken message is delivered from a physician to a patient that is crucial to the development of their relationship, and that determines whether or not the ensuing relationship will have positive or negative consequences for the participants. Those physicians who develop rapport and trust with patients, who exhibit positive attitudes toward them and who inspire confidence in their patients about their recommendations for treatment are more likely to be busy and successful physicians. What a physician actually says to the patient during the patient visit may be less important to the patient than the process and the tone of the total physician–patient visit with the doctor. Successful and aware physicians recognize that their communication and interpersonal skills are just as important as their clinical skills.

In addition to communication and interpersonal skills, medical students, residents and practicing physicians must also understand how important good writing skills are to the transfer of effective and important clinical information as an accompaniment to effective patient care. It is a disservice to patients for physicians to make brilliant diagnoses only to garble the information in subsequent letters to referring physicians. Improved writing skills can be developed by physicians, but only if they are willing to make a conscious and determined effort to improve their writing skills as an additional form of physician communication. Improvement in writing skills begins with developing the ability to transfer medical information to readers and to other physicians clearly, in simple terms, and in a form that is easily grasped and understood by other physicians and readers. Like all acquired skills, a physician's ability to communicate well with patients, and to write effectively, requires a lot of practice and a will to succeed. Once physicians have developed their skills in communicating effectively with patients, and in writing clearly and succinctly for readers, they will then be well on their way to becoming better and more effective physician communicators.

Chapter 9

# Improved Physician Interpersonal Skills

The medical profession regards communication and interpersonal skills as necessary qualifications for physicians to possess. The ability to interact successfully with patients and others is regarded as a necessity for physicians if they are to be able to provide good medical care for patients, and it is an acknowledged goal of good medical education. Despite this professed importance, gaining proficiency in these skills has been given little prominence in the traditional medical school curriculum, particularly by comparison with the time and emphasis given to biotechnology by medical schools. Although physicians' communication skills have been found to be related to clinical outcomes and patient satisfaction, teaching of communication skills has not been fully integrated into many medical school curricula or adequately evaluated with large-scale controlled trials.[19]

As a consequence, many medical schools produce new physicians each year who continue to display a lack of balance between an emphasis on curing and an emphasis on caring. Although empathy is recognizable in those physicians who possess this quality, empirical investigations of patient empathy are scarce because of conceptual ambiguity and the lack of a psychometrically sound tool for measuring physician empathy. Although empathy cannot yet be accurately measured from a scientific viewpoint, most sick patients can instinctively recognize which physicians display empathy toward them and which do not.

Another vital element of effective medical communication is clarity in the written and spoken material that physicians produce. Confused writing and speaking by physicians can be a danger to patients and others because it lends itself to misinterpretation and misunderstanding of its intended meaning. The content material of what physicians say or write must be clearly constructed and must be presented to others in such a manner that it can be easily and completely understood by listening and reading audiences. Communication with patients and others is both an interaction and a process based on a background of human behavior and social science research, and is defined by a specific body of knowledge. Although the activity encompassed by physician–patient communication includes the transmitting and imparting of medical information, the process of physician–patient communication is a dynamic one that goes beyond the simple transmitting of a message or the imparting of information to others. The communication process is in a constant state of change in that its content material is influenced by the environment and by the situation in which the communication takes place, as well as by the relationships that exist between the communicating participants. Perception of the quality of the medical care delivered to patients by physicians depends to a great extent on the assessment by patients of the quality of the human communication developed between them and their physicians.

A study of the Medicare program by the Institute of Medicine in Washington, DC in 1990 listed several deficiencies at that time in the practice behaviors of physicians, including poor relationships with patients. This study highlighted the recognition that medical care has to become a type of mutual participation activity in which health care decisions are believed to be a responsibility properly shared between physicians and patients. This view makes it even more important that physicians function as patient advocates and that they practice medicine more as teachers of patients, and less as authority figures. To be able to teach patients effectively, physicians must be able to communicate with them in clear and understandable language so as to elicit their full cooperation and understanding in the management of their particular medical problems. Unfortunately, some practicing physicians believe themselves to be too busy or too important to spend much time communicating with sick patients. After all, too many physicians seem to believe that this is what medical assistants and residents are for.

Long gone are the days when physicians were the sole providers of medical information to both patients and the public. Health and wellness are topics of great interest to both patients and the general public, and physicians no longer seem to be the primary sources of such information for patients. The mass media now provides health information and health education material in large quantities, and physicians need to accept the responsibility of ensuring that their patients understand that the health information provided by the mass media is not always accurate. In addition, most of today's patients seem to have lost their previously held awe of physicians, and no longer believe that questioning their physician about medical decisions implies a lack of confidence in them. There is simply too much public information available to patients about medical treatment options, and physicians need to recognize that the old saying ''doctor knows best'' is now long out of date. A large measure of patient dissatisfaction and patient resentment arising from clinical encounters with physicians originates because some physicians tend to respond to these patient attitudes in a careless, thoughtless or insensitive fashion. Regardless of cause or origin, insensitivity of physicians toward patients is a serious deterrent to the development of effective communication with them.

It is neither appropriate nor possible to give thoughtful and effective medical care to patients in a quick or offhand fashion, or by delegating this medical responsibility to someone else. Patients want and need to discuss their medical problems and concerns with their chosen physician, and they have every right to expect that this will happen. Communication nightmares in these patient–physician interactions can be lessened by teaching all health care professionals involved, including physicians, the reasons for accepting their roles as patient advocates and patient teachers, and by structuring the clinical encounter and its environment so that the primary goal of the effort is not physician convenience, but rather the improved outcome of medical treatment from a patient's viewpoint. The general attitude and atmosphere of a physician's office or other outpatient site must be set by the physician in charge, the primary goal being the achievement of more efficient and effective medical care.

The overriding goal of good physician–patient communication is to improve the outcome of provided patient care from the patient's point of view. Outcomes of diagnosis and treatment will depend greatly on unimpaired communication between physician and patient. Failure to establish empathic relationships with patients can be a serious bar to good communication and effective patient responses. The quality of medical care rendered in the physician–patient interaction depends greatly on the interaction between physicians and patients, and the suspicion remains that these interactions, more often than they should be, are disappointing to both parties in the clinical encounter. There may be insensitive communication between physicians and patients for multiple reasons, and the fault may lie with either party.

Patients can be demanding, querulous, hostile, suspicious, exceedingly sensitive and highly dependent. However, much of the patient dissatisfaction and unhappiness that arises from clinical encounters with physicians is due to the fact that physicians may respond to their patients' projected attitudes in a careless, thoughtless or insensitive fashion. Regardless of its cause or origin, insensitivity toward a patient's declared symptoms or health problems is a major deterrent to the development of effective communication between physician and patient. Patients should not have to drag information about their health problem from their physician. Those physicians who treat patients with respect and attention and who have recognized the need to master the skills and techniques of good communication are more likely to gather full and accurate information from patients, to dispense clear and persuasive information to them and their families, and to elicit cooperation and acceptance of the details of patient management from patients and others involved in the process of dispensing good medical care.

Chapter 10

# Physicians' Voices

Physicians' voices are vital to the practice of good medical care because they can be used to inspire hope and comfort in sick and desperately ill patients. Physician voices, when used appropriately, can inspire and lift the spirits of very sick patients, even when hope for their survival is extremely limited. Before any offered professional advice can be followed for benefit, the physician's voice must be understood clearly by patients, by listeners at medical meetings, and by readers of published medical articles. Messages delivered to patients and to medical audiences by physicians should be well conceived, deliberate, concise and correct. After choosing medicine as a career, physicians face additional choices about career options and opportunities for service. A popular and clearly visible option for service lies in treating the injured and healing the sick, but other options also exist. Combined with a clinical career, or as an independent option, physicians may elect to teach in order to share their knowledge and expertise with medical students, residents and other physicians. Some physicians may seek a career in medical research in order to contribute to the scientific knowledge base that supports clinical decision making. Regardless of the choice that is made, these differing career paths and opportunities for service are bound together by a common thread of effective written and spoken communication on the part of the physician. To receive, record and transmit medical information accurately, succinctly and with clarity is a skill that is basic to the practice of every branch of medicine, and one that all physicians should strive hard to possess, no matter which medical career path they have chosen. Good physician communicators recognize that effective communication with patients and others is the key to medical success, and they know that knowledge combined with effective communication skills is a powerful tool for any physician to possess.

Human communication is believed to be the physician's single most important skill for providing good and effective medical care to sick patients, because of the ability of good physician communication skills to lessen fear and to relieve anxiety in patients. This belief underscores the importance of the need for physicians to strive to develop effective medical writing and verbal communication skills for use in their professional careers. The ability to communicate effectively with readers, listeners, patients and others in need of health-related information and health advice is both a skill and an art. However, the available evidence supports the suspicion that many physicians are at present deficient in both the skill and the art of effective communication with patients and others.

Unfortunately, little assessment of or even education in medical writing or communication skills is currently provided in the curricula of most medical schools and in most graduate medical education programs in this country. Rather, these most desirable physician skills are left to be learned in a rather hit-or-miss fashion by medical students and residents, mainly through personal initiative.

Communication between and among humans is an interaction as well as a process based upon a background of human behavior and social science research, and is defined by a body of identifiable knowledge. The word "communication" derives from a Greek root meaning "to bring together." Although the activity encompassed by communication includes the transmitting and imparting of information, the action involved in bringing people together for the sharing of information is an active process that goes beyond the passive activity implied by simply transmitting information. The sharing of information in an effective communication process initiates changes in the behavior, thinking, lifestyle and attitude of those receiving the information. A communication process achieves its full potential when appropriate relationships exist or are developed between the communicator, the message and the recipient of the message. Communication is an interaction or relationship between humans that involves the production of a written or spoken message and the receipt of that message by someone else. It is this ongoing process of sending and receiving messages that results in the creation of a positive or negative communication relationship between humans, which depends to a great extent on the content matter of the delivered message.

It is often the manner or style in which a spoken message is delivered from a physician to a patient that is crucial for the development of their relationship and for determining whether or not the ensuing relationship will develop positive or negative connotations for the participants. It is in the interview process with new patients in particular that physicians are expected to obtain the patient-related information needed for them to take the actions necessary to diagnose and treat the problems that are being experienced by the patients. A primary goal for physicians when conducting new patient interviews should be to obtain sufficient information from them in a pleasant and efficient manner to enable a proper and correct diagnosis to be approached or determined, and an appropriate patient management program or treatment program to be agreed upon.

There also is reason to believe that the effective use of language has a persuasive dimension in that one cannot communicate at all without making some effort to persuade the recipient of the communicated message in one way or another. All communication behavior has as its purpose the elicitation of a specific response from a particular person or a group of people. Therefore in order to become more effective communicators, physicians first need to understand the underlying purpose of communicating with patients and others by either the spoken or written word. Effective communication with patients and others involves more skills than merely giving a message that is not infrequently delivered in a stern authoritarian tone and in a time frame just short of being rude.

The medical profession has a particularly persuasive claim to authority, which must be respected but not abused by its practitioners. Physicians come into direct and intimate contact with all types of people in their daily lives. They are present at births and at deaths, and at other transitional moments of daily living, and they interpret people's interpersonal problems in the language of scientific knowledge. Physicians have the ability to offer a kind of individualized objectivity and a personal relationship with sick patients that has the potential to inspire confidence in these patients. The very nature of sickness or serious injury tends to promote acceptance in patients of their physician's recommendations for treatment. Physicians in turn have a professional obligation to provide competent, compassionate and empathic medical care for patients. Good communication skills therefore promote a relationship between physician and patient that facilitates care of the illness or injury, enhances patient self-reliance, and helps to ensure that all of the relevant issues will be brought to bear on the diagnostic and therapeutic process. This can be accomplished to its fullest extent by those physicians who can develop rapport and trust with patients, who can instill confidence in patients that recommended procedures and treatments are in their best interests, and who exhibit positive attitudes toward people. Effective medical communication allows the exchange of thoughts, ideas, data, conclusions and other types of information to bring about beneficial changes between physician communicators, patients and other audiences.

It is in the interview process with new patients that physicians are expected to obtain the patient-related information required for them to take the appropriate actions necessary to diagnose and treat the medical problem for which the patient is seeking help. Under no circumstances should the patient interview be rushed, because an extra five minutes during the patient interview might well disclose the extra information critical to a correct diagnosis. The interviewing doctor should be confident, empathic, humane, personal, forthright, respectful and thorough. Vocal repetition is not a widely admired personal attribute in most people, except in medical care situations. Doctors who advise patients on health issues frequently need to repeat their medical instructions in order to ensure patient understanding and compliance.

For patient interviews to be successful, physicians need to possess appropriate communication skills in order to question patients appropriately and carefully, and to listen to their responses attentively so that the maximum amount of patient information can be elicited during the patient interview process.

Physicians will gain more information from patients if they project genuine concern for the patient and his or her medical problem, and if they ask their questions in a gently persuasive tone of voice rather than by using an authoritative tone and medical jargon. Patient interview outcomes will be improved if physicians provide patients with sufficient time and encouragement to describe their medical problem adequately, rather than leading them along with short-answer questions and frequent interruptions in order to hasten the interview process. When structuring interviews, physicians must schedule enough time for the patient visit so that patients are satisfied that they had sufficient time to tell their medical story to the doctor. Giving patients a more active role in the interview process has been shown to have positive consequences in that patients are better able to express their needs, articulate their concerns, and cooperate with physician recommendations about diagnosis and suggested treatment. Patients' perceptions of their selected physician's warmth and understanding also correlate positively with their being able to talk about their medical problem in their own words during the physician interview. Obtaining objective information about their illness, the proposed treatment plan and their prognosis from the interviewing physician is rated by patients as being extremely important.

The most successful physician interviews from a patient perspective are patient centered as opposed to physician centered. Good patient-centered physician interviews combine a careful analysis of the patient's symptoms and physical signs with an understanding by the physician of the patient's concerns about their medical problem and the implications that it might have for their future health. This type of patient interview is most successful when combined with the interpersonal skills of listening, observing and responding on the part of the involved physician. A patient-centered interview recognizes and acknowledges the patient as a person with a unique life history and a special set of needs which happen to be accompanying a medical problem for which the patient is seeking help. Physicians who are skilled at conducting patient-centered interviews are generally able to obtain more pertinent information from patients about their medical problems than are physicians who are not so skilled.

Physicians who are experts in establishing rapport and trust with patients are more likely to be characterized as open-minded and flexible by patients, and are more likely to exhibit positive attitudes toward patients. Insightful and sensitive physicians have learned how to interpret and respond to the nuances of both verbal and non-verbal communication exchanges between patients and themselves. The ability to establish rapport and trust with patients must also include the physician's ability and willingness to deal with intimate emotional material associated with patients and, on occasion, with patients' families. Unfortunately, some physicians tend to try to avoid dealing with intimate patient material because of their own personal discomfort with such patient conversations or interactions. However, sensitive and caring physicians approach emotion-laden clinical encounters with patients with the understanding that empathy is the physician's vital tool for understanding the patient and their medical problem. Empathic physicians also recognize the differing effects on sick patients of pity, sympathy and empathy. Pity rarely helps sick and distressed patients, sympathy frequently helps them, but empathy always helps them.

As applied to the physician–patient interaction, empathy is the feeling relationship that can develop when the physician clearly understands the patient's medical problem as if he himself or she herself was the patient, and recognizes the medical problem and its impact on the patient through the eyes of the patient. An empathic physician can identify with a sick patient yet at the same time can maintain sufficient professional detachment to be able to make appropriate clinical decisions on behalf of that patient. Physicians who do not or cannot develop empathic relationships with patients tend to maintain a more rigid distance from their patients in the unsubstantiated belief that this attitude of detachment strengthens their image as authority figures and increases their power to reassure their patients. Human beings are designed by evolution to form meaningful interpersonal relationships through verbal and non-verbal communication. Neither a physician's depth of knowledge nor their interviewing skills will be sufficient to provide effective and compassionate medical care unless the physician's behavior and attitude during the clinical encounter convey to the patient the sense that, for the physician, addressing the patient's medical problem ranks above all other considerations in the interview process. Empathy for sick patients, combined with a positive attitude toward helping them to regain their health, is the mark of a true physician healer. Being regarded by patients as a true physician healer and as a good physician communicator are goals that all physicians should strive to attain.

# Appendix

## Technical Writing Should be Taught in Medical Schools

When I discussed my planned retirement from clinical medicine with our University President in late 1993, he countered by asking me to become Thomas Jefferson University's first medical editor. I soon found myself in a very small one-room office with a new computer, but no secretary or other office help. This new editorial service was developed to be voluntary and was available free of charge as a help to potential authors from the institution's School of Medicine, University Hospital, Bluemle Cancer Center, Farber Neurological Institute, Wills Eye Hospital, and the College of Graduate Studies. Since the opening of this office in late 1993, I have had the opportunity to review and edit about 960 submitted manuscripts written for possible publication to date.

This editing experience to date has strengthened my observation that most initial writing efforts in medicine and in basic science are not focused properly on the principal goal of medical and basic science writing which should be the reader of the profferred information. In many manuscript submissions it seems clearly apparent that the reader was given little thought or consideration. Most potential authors interviewed in this office were completely uninformed about the important technical differences between literary writing and technical writing in constructing manuscripts for possible publication in medical and basic science journals. It seems apparent that most initial writing efforts in medicine and basic science are poorly done because most medical and basic science authors are uninformed about the critical differences between literary writing and technical writing in constructing manuscripts for possible publication. It seems quite apparent from all the criticism leveled at the writing skills of physicians and basic scientists that marked improvement in these skills would be welcomed and should be a useful goal for all of us to try to attain. While some writing experts believe that literary writing ability cannot be taught, others believe that technical writing can be learned as a skill. It is, then, the further development of technical writing skills in physicians to which much more attention needs to be paid by teaching these required skills in medical schools.

Writing courses for medical students can be simple in design and limited in scope and emphasis if most medical educators will accept the view that medical writing is a form of technical writing and, as such, differs markedly in purpose and style from literary and creative writing. Medical writing can be taught as a form of technical writing in medical schools, with the principal teaching effort focused on medical students learning how to express themselves in the crisp and lean style of good medical writing. Teaching technical writing in medical schools should focus on the seven writing tasks carried out most frequently by physicians in their professional careers:

1  writing office medical records
2  writing letters to referring physicians
3  writing patient histories and physical examinations
4  writing progress notes
5  writing discharge summaries
6  writing peer reviewed medical articles
7  writing grant proposals.

While these tasks represent important, complex, and different writing purposes which physicians carry out with varying degrees of frequency, or infrequency, it appears that most medical schools do not offer medical students formal instruction on how to perform these writing tasks. Courses developed to teach writing skills to medical students should be designed with the primary intent of teaching medical students how to express themselves clearly and correctly in written form, and should focus their teaching emphasis on the above seven writing tasks which physicians carry out most frequently in their professional careers. In addition, opportunities for medical students to practice and sharpen their writing skills should be woven into the fabric of the entire medical education experience.

Medical writing courses, in addition to reviewing with students the fundamentals of grammar, syntax, and sentence structure, and trying to develop in them a facility for the use of the English language, should concentrate on teaching future physicians how to achieve clarity, accuracy, precision, logic, and discipline in their writing efforts. Physicians use logical sequencing in arriving at diagnostic conclusions and treatment plans, and their written material should reflect appropriate use of the English language presented to readers in similarly derived logically written sequences. The criticisms leveled at the writing efforts of some physicians and medical scientists make it imperative that marked improvement in these skills be a necessary goal to attempt to achieve. While some writing experts believe that writing ability cannot be taught, others, including this author, believe that technical writing can be learned as a skill, and it is to the further development of the skill of technical writing that more attention needs to be paid in medical schools.

If future physicians are to be regarded as more sensitive and empathic toward their patients as fellow human beings, and are to be regarded as more attentive to their medical care needs, medical schools will have to give greater emphasis to the nurturing of appropriate physician attitudes and behaviors toward patients and to the development of better physician communication and interpersonal skills.[20] Positive educational efforts must begin early in the effort to educate medical students and should extend throughout the entire medical education process in order to teach and enhance the humanistic interpersonal and communicating skills of future physicians. If these latter qualities are to be valued and emphasized in medical practitioners, they must be taught, nourished, and kept in proper balance throughout the entire course of medical school education.[21] In addition to gaining medical knowledge and learning clinical medical skills in medical school, future physicians must learn a set of appropriate behaviors and attitudes which will serve to connect the physicians' professional, scholarly, and personal preparation for medical careers with the patients they are learning to serve.

The practice of modern medicine is a complicated mixture of demands because it is both a highly technical healing science and a more amorphous healing art which must be practiced with compassion, concern, and appropriate respect for fellow human beings who become sick or injured. In order for future physicians to be most effective in this more socially aware practice environment, medical educators must include in their curricula instructions these effective components of good patient care. These are extra demands to place on medical students, but they need to understand how important this aspect of medical practice will be to them if they aspire to satisfying professional careers. Medical school curricula should be modified to provide medical students with the understanding and tools to address these important patient needs and the skills of technical writing while, at the same time, maintaining their own professional effectiveness.

# Bibliography

1 Gartland JJ. Practice guidelines for orthopaedics. In: Mann RD, Vallance-Owen AJ, editors. *Medical Audit and Accountability*. London: International Congress and Symposium Series, Royal Society of Medicine Services; 1992.

2 Woods D. *Communication for Doctors. How to Improve Patient Care and Minimise Legal Risks*. Oxford: Radcliffe Publishing; 2004.

3 Schwager E. *Medical English. Usage and Abusage*. Phoenix, AZ: Oryx Press; 1991.

4 Lang TA. Medical writing is not one of the humanities. *Am Med Writers Assoc J*. 1987; **2(5):** 3–8.

5 White EB. *The Elements of Style*. New York: The Macmillan Company; 1959.

6 Byrne DW. *Publishing Your Medical Research Paper*. Baltimore, MD: Williams & Wilkins; 1998.

7 Williams JM. *Style. Ten Lessons in Clarity and Grace*. Glenview, IL: Scott, Foresman and Company; 1957.

8 Huth EJ. *Medical Style and Format. An International Manual for Authors, Editors and Publishers*. Philadelphia, PA: ISI Press; 1987.

9 Woodford FP, editor. *Scientific Writing for Graduate Students. A Manual on the Teaching of Scientific Writing*. Bethesda, MD: Council of Biology Editors, Committee on Graduate Training in Scientific Writing; 1986.

10 Gastel B. *Presenting Science to the Public*. Philadelphia, PA: ISI Press; 1983.

11 Staheli LT. *Speaking and Writing for the Physician*. New York: Raven Press; 1986.

12 Gitlin LM, Lyons KJ. *Successful Grant Writing. Strategies for Health and Human Services Professionals*. 2nd ed. New York: Springer Publishing Company; 2004.

13 Eaves GN. Who reads your project grant application to the National Institutes of Health? *Fed Proc*. 1972; **31:** 7–10.

14 DeBakey L. The persuasive proposal. *J Tech Writing Commun*. 1976; **6:** 17–21.

15 Hojat M. *Empathy in Patient Care: Antecedents, Development, Measurement and Outcomes*. New York: Springer Publishing Company; 2006.

16 Ludmerer KM. *Time to Heal*. New York: Oxford University Press; 1999.

17 Halpern J. *From Detached Concern to Sympathy. Humanizing Medical Practice*. New York: Oxford University Press; 2001.

18 Street RL, Gordon HS, Ward MM *et al*. Patient participation in medical

consultations: why some patients are more involved than others. *Med Care.* 2005; **43:** 960–69.

19 Yedidia MJ, Gillespie CC, Kacher E *et al.* Effect of communication training on medical student performance. *JAMA.* 2003; **290:** 1157–65.

20 Gartland JJ. *Medical Writing and Communicating.* Frederick, MD: University Publishing Group; 1993, pp. 223–8.

21 Federman DD. The education of medical students: sounds, alarums, and excursions. *Acad Med.* 1990; **65(4):** 221–6.

# Index